Still Me

Praise for *Still Me*

'A beautifully written, personal, empathetic and immensely practical book. Sabina illuminates the path in front of us, wherever we are on this journey'

– Dr Harry Barry, GP, author and mental health advocate

'*Still Me* speaks directly to what matters to people like me – living with dementia but still very much here. It echoes our truths, respects our voices and reminds the world that we are still living, still growing and still ourselves'

– Helen Rochford-Brennan, Global Dementia Ambassador

'A wonderful resource for any family affected by dementia'

– Judy Williams, The Alzheimer Society of Ireland

'Dr Sabina Brennan's compassionate approach and deep level of understanding of the care partner's lived experience gives us back our sense of self, gives us solace, and it fills us with hope for the journey ahead'

– Helena Quaid, Chair, Dementia Carers Campaign Network

'Sabina understands how important the partnership is between caregiver and dementia patient, and draws on the most up-to-date and innovative research to show how to both optimise the caregiving experience and boost wellbeing and brain health for both. A long-overdue resource'

– Kim Tully, Chief Executive, Engaging Dementia

'A comprehensive resource for care-givers. The dementia journey takes everyone with it. It can be hugely challenging, but also hugely rewarding. It places significant mental and physical pressures on care-givers so self-care is essential for all parties. It's great to see these simple tips laid out here for readers to adopt in their own lives'

– Dr Julia Jones, neuroscientist

'A compassionate and insightful guide for anyone supporting a loved one with dementia ... What truly sets this book apart is its positive and encouraging tone. Sabina deeply understands the emotional and physical demands on care partners and emphasises the importance of self-care and support. It's filled with actionable, real-world tips that can make a genuine difference in day-to-day life'

– Catherine O'Keeffe, menopause coach and founder of Wellness Warrior

Dr Sabina Brennan

Still Me

A neuroscientist's guide to caring for someone with dementia

GREEN TREE
LONDON · OXFORD · NEW YORK · NEW DELHI · SYDNEY

GREEN TREE
Bloomsbury Publishing Plc
50 Bedford Square, London, WC1B 3DP, UK
Bloomsbury Publishing Ireland Limited,
29 Earlsfort Terrace, Dublin 2, D02 AY28, Ireland

BLOOMSBURY, GREEN TREE and the Green Tree logo are trademarks of Bloomsbury Publishing Plc

First published in Great Britain 2025

Copyright © Sabina Brennan 2025

Sabina Brennan has asserted her right under the Copyright, Designs and Patents Act, 1988, to be identified as Author of this work.

Every reasonable effort has been made to trace copyright holders of material reproduced in this book, but if any have been inadvertently overlooked the publishers would be glad to hear from them. For legal purposes the Acknowledgements on p. 283 constitute an extension of this copyright page.

All rights reserved. No part of this publication may be: i) reproduced or transmitted in any form, electronic or mechanical, including photocopying, recording or by means of any information storage or retrieval system without prior permission in writing from the publishers; or ii) used or reproduced in any way for the training, development or operation of artificial intelligence (AI) technologies, including generative AI technologies. The rights holders expressly reserve this publication from the text and data mining exception as per Article 4(3) of the Digital Single Market Directive (EU) 2019/790

Bloomsbury Publishing Plc does not have any control over, or responsibility for, any third-party websites referred to or in this book. All internet addresses given in this book were correct at the time of going to press. The author and publisher regret any inconvenience caused if addresses have changed or sites have ceased to exist but can accept no responsibility for any such changes.

A catalogue record for this book is available from the British Library.

Library of Congress Cataloguing-in-Publication data has been applied for.

ISBN: HB: 978-1-3994-2138-6; eBook: 978-1399-42142-3; ePDF: 978-1-3994-2143-0

2 4 6 8 10 9 7 5 3 1

Typeset in IBM Plex Serif by Deanta Global Publishing Services, Chennai, India
Printed and bound in Great Britain by CPI Group (UK) Ltd, Croydon, CR0 4YY

MIX
Paper | Supporting responsible forestry
FSC
www.fsc.org   FSC® C013604

To find out more about our authors and books visit www.bloomsbury.com and sign up for our newsletters.
For product safety related questions contact productsafety@bloomsbury.com

For those who care

Still Me

I have dementia and I am still me
When I am confused and frightened
Hold me close, calm my heart, and still me.

I care for you and I am still me
When my patience wears thin and I ache to be free
When I wish for you to be you and me to be me,
I'll pause, breathe deep, and let our love still me.

Together we walk through fog and stormy sea,
Bound by our love and the truth that
You are still you and I am still me.

– Dr Sabina Brennan

Contents

Introduction	8
Section One: Self-care	**13**
1. Burden	17
2. Health	46
3. Stress	67
4. Support	87
5. Coping	99
6. Reward	108
Section Two: Still Me	**123**
7. See me	125
8. Understand me	159
Section Three: Live Well	**181**
9. Making the most of what you've got	183
10. Minimising the tough stuff	198
11. Maximising the good stuff	245
Appendix	277
References	278
Acknowledgements	283
Index	286

Introduction

Dementia is devastating. Not just for the person diagnosed but also for their family. But it's not the end of the world. There is life after diagnosis. In fact, it is possible for you and the person that you care for to live well and even enjoy life with dementia. *Still Me*, aimed at family care partners, will help you to do just that.

I use the term 'care partner' throughout this book rather than the more usual terms of carer or caregiver. I do this for two reasons. First, an individual living with dementia needs someone who sees them as a person, an equal and a partner. Someone who will support their independence, not take it away by doing things for them. They need a care partner who will help them to live the best life they can for as long as possible. Second, when we see ourselves as carers or caregivers, while meaning well and acting out of love and a desire to protect, we can inadvertently and unintentionally place ourselves in a position of power and may do things that disempower the person we care for, and in so doing accelerate the progression of their dementia.

Care partners can be spouses, life partners, children, siblings, friends or other relatives. For ease, I generally refer to the person with dementia as your relative but please take that to include you, whatever your relationship is to the person with dementia. Care partners can be part-time, full-time, living with or separately from the person with dementia. Even if your relative is living in a care home or has some professional care at home, you are still a care partner if you support the person with dementia in some way.

Whether you are just starting your journey as a care partner and are still reeling from the diagnosis, or have been on the journey for a very long time and are running out of steam, I hope you will find something in this practical book to make life better for you and for your relative with dementia. I know from personal experience when my own mum was diagnosed that it can be really challenging to think clearly, let alone think about self-care. Caring for a relative with dementia is incredibly demanding, both psychologically and physically. When dementia arrives in your life, it doesn't come with extra hours, extra energy or the extra headspace you need to come to terms with the diagnosis, make decisions AND meet the everyday and ever-increasing demands of providing care. Dementia arrived in my life at a time when an ongoing stressful situation at work was impacting significantly on my health and a difficult boss was placing unreasonable demands on my time. I totally understand how the idea of self-care might feel like just another task on an already overloaded to-do list.

Tucked within these pages, therefore, you will find strategies, ideas and advice for self-care in a way that is achievable and makes you feel supported rather than overwhelmed and further burdened. I hope that by framing self-care as an integral and necessary part of caregiving, you will begin to see it as an essential recharge, a way to renew your batteries, an energy source rather than an energy-draining demand. Many of the suggestions I share to help you sustain your energy and emotional well-being over the long term can be integrated into your existing daily routines. Even micro-moments of self-care that take only a minute or two can make a significant difference in protecting your health and preventing burnout.

If any of my pleas for you to see self-care as essential rather than optional come across as rigid demands, please remember that my intention is to help, not to hinder. Self-care is flexible and personal. There is no 'right way' to do it. What matters is that you feel supported. You can adapt the self-care practices within these pages to fit your preferences, your daily schedule, your life. It's OK to feel overwhelmed. You are doing enough. Taking a moment to yourself is not neglectful or weak but rather an act of courage and sustainability.

I am acutely aware that when I write about the importance of core elements of self-care – such as stress management, sleep, nutrition and social connection – and highlight the negative impacts their lack can have on your health and well-being, it can make for depressing reading. Try not to get too hung up on the negative aspects of this information; instead, try to reframe it as a motivator. Think of getting enough sleep, healthy eating and connecting with people socially as a simplified framework for self-care. If you could manage just these three things then you are winning in the self-care stakes.

I offer lots of tips for assistive technology and resources that may provide support and allow you to enjoy crucial breaks. You don't have to adopt them all, or indeed any of them if none feel like a good fit. Choose only the technology and other resources that feel right for you on your personal caring journey.

Learning to set boundaries is key to successful self-care. This is something I struggled with when caring for Mum. If, like me, you struggle to say 'no' in other areas of your life, the prospect of learning to ask for help and to prioritise your well-being to benefit you and your relative might seem daunting, but approach it with resolve and you will find the payoff is well worth it. I was surprised to learn that saying 'no' didn't result in negative consequences. In fact, I felt huge relief and a sense of achievement when I said no or when I asked for help. I didn't feel like a failure and I didn't feel guilty.

My aim is to show you that self-care is a vital, yet manageable, component of caregiving. I want you to see it as a source of strength and support for both you and your relative. I hope this book helps you to view self-care not as an indulgence but as a necessary and compassionate act of self-preservation.

I hope the anecdotes about life with dementia in the chapters that follow will resonate with you. They reflect common experiences as well as my personal experience of caring for my mum, who lived with dementia. In my professional capacity as a psychologist and neuroscientist, my expertise lies in the area of brain health, dementia risk reduction, dementia and dementia caregiving. I had the privilege of directing a dementia research programme at Trinity College Dublin, where my research included examining the impact that caregiving has on spouses. I also led Brain Fit, a comprehensive project exploring the intricate relationship between brain health, lifestyle, genomics and dementia risk. My journey in this field has been driven by a deep commitment to understanding and advocating for those affected by dementia and other neurological conditions. This commitment extends beyond academia; I have actively contributed to several national and global advocacy committees and advisory boards, offering guidance and insight to shape policy and improve care practices.

My work has also involved advising both the Irish government and the All Party Parliamentary Group on Longevity in the United Kingdom, bringing attention to the urgent needs surrounding dementia care and dementia risk reduction. Additionally, I have been a vocal advocate in the media, shedding light on the many challenges faced by individuals with dementia and their care partners.

Recognising the importance of practical, accessible information grounded in science, I have developed award-winning materials including an app, websites and animations. These tools have been translated into multiple languages, to help people to understand dementia, care for people with dementia, boost brain health, reduce the risk of developing dementia and support those caring for a relative living with dementia. The societal impact of my efforts has been acknowledged through several awards, underscoring my dedication to making a meaningful difference in the lives of people affected by dementia.

The book has three sections:

Section 1: Self-care
The book begins by focusing on you, the care partner. Using scientific research and examples, I explain the factors that can influence whether your role as a care partner has a positive or negative impact on your health and well-being. By completing questionnaires, you will gain important insight into your own experience. These insights, together with my practical tips, will help you to make adjustments to reduce your stress levels, improve your health, develop useful coping strategies and reap the positive benefits of being a care partner. Benefits that are all too easy to miss in the midst of a life-changing dementia diagnosis.

Section 2: Still Me
This section switches focus from you to your relative. The information in this section will help you to better understand your relative's symptoms. There is no point in sugar-coating the fact that some symptoms can be very challenging. My aim is to arm you with knowledge and practical advice to

help you to reduce the incidence of challenging symptoms and deal with those that you do encounter with minimal impact on your health and well-being and that of your relative. Once you have a good understanding of the disease, the aim really is to help you to focus on the person rather than their disease. Developing dementia won't stop your relative from wanting the same things we all want – happiness, enjoyment and love. All of these are still possible once you shift focus from the disease to the person.

Section 3: Live Well
This section outlines evidence-based therapies that can be used in the early stages of dementia to stimulate cognition and restore functional ability in ways that add meaning and improve quality of life. There are practical tips on dementia-specific communication to help you to sustain meaningful interactions with your relative while you support their independence and enable their ongoing engagement with life. There is also clear information to help you to understand and manage neuropsychiatric symptoms and other behaviours that can be a challenge. The final chapter in this section is full of ideas to adopt a brain-healthy lifestyle for your personal well-being that, if also adopted by your relative, may slow progression of their symptoms. There are simple strategies, memory aids, as well as tips on supportive technology and making your home dementia friendly.

At the end of each section, you will find a summary of the key points and practical tips from each chapter.

SECTION 1
Self-care

Self-care isn't self-indulgent, it's good judgement

A good carer puts the person they care for first and puts their own needs on hold, right? Wrong. On an aeroplane, there's a reason you're told to put your own oxygen mask on first before helping others. Self-care isn't self-indulgent – it's good judgement. When your needs are taken care of, the person you support will benefit too. We know from research that a person providing dementia care can experience negative effects on their own health and overall well-being. The advice within these pages is designed to help you to maintain good health and a good quality of life while you provide care. Dementia care requires stamina: the journey is more a marathon than a sprint. It doesn't make sense to allow your health to suffer as a consequence of caring. The last thing you want is a situation where you are too ill to care for your relative. The best thing, in what really is a difficult situation, is to try to be sensible and realistic about the amount of quality care you can personally provide. When we are under stress, it's hard to see things clearly or logically. Sometimes, others can see the problem more easily, so seek and listen to advice.

In the initial stages, you may find there is a good match between what you can provide and what your relative needs. However, as the disease progresses you may need professional care services. Taking advantage of state-provided care services – or employing a professional carer from a private company, if you can afford it – is a great way to preserve your health and your relationship with your relative. Organisations like the Alzheimer's Society provide life-changing support and services. Their online family carer training can help you to understand what is going on with your relative and offer advice on how to cope. Further along in the disease, Alzheimer's Society day-care centres can make the world of difference.

Research indicates that a person with dementia who is supported at home has a better quality of life and more positive outcomes than a person with dementia who lives in residential care. Having said that it is important to bear in mind that the relationship between living arrangements and quality of life for a person with dementia is complex. Factors such as the quality of care provided, opportunities for social engagement and the preferences of individuals play crucial roles. While some studies indicate potential benefits of home-based care, others highlight the challenges and stressors faced by family care partners, which can impact both the care partner and the person with dementia's well-being. While home-based care for individuals with dementia may offer certain advantages in terms of their quality of life any decisions made between home care and residential care must be personalised to the specific situation and context. Decisions need to consider the person with dementia's specific needs, the health and well-being of their care partner, availability of support systems and the quality of care that can be provided in either setting.

I want to make it very clear that support at home doesn't need to be provided by one person – it can come from multiple family members sharing the caring, or a combination of relatives and professional services, or indeed full-time professional care provided in the person's own home. This is very important information to take on board, especially if you have significant health challenges yourself, are at a later stage of life where you lack the strength or stamina to meet your relative's care needs, have other commitments or have sufficient self-awareness to acknowledge that you are not the best person to provide care for your relative. Remember, providing the best possible care for your relative doesn't mean you have to provide that care personally. Nor does it mean you have to drop everything or change your life completely to provide all of that care yourself. Depending on your age, your health and other circumstances, external support such as in-home professional care, residential care, day care or a combination may be the only viable option (see page 38 for tips and advice on choosing professional care).

The key is to find a balance between maintaining and protecting your own health and ensuring that your relative has a good quality of life. This often means making compromises and finding creative solutions that support your relative and ensure you both enjoy good health. There is no magic recipe; it is a delicate balance and the compromises and solutions that are right for you will be contingent on multiple factors such as your age, any health conditions you may have, your finances, your job, your commitments, your relative's symptoms and the stage of the disease. These factors will change over time, so you will need to constantly re-evaluate your decisions and choices and make adjustments according to evolving circumstances. Caring for a relative full-time at home isn't a feasible option for everyone, and even if it is possible to care for your relative at home in the early stages, this may change as the disease and associated symptoms and demands change. Towards the end, it may be in your relative's best interests to move to a facility where there is access to the medical and other support your relative will need as they come to the end of their journey. So please don't feel bad or guilty if your relative is cared for in a care home rather than at home. My mum lived in a care home for the last few years of her life.

While I knew she would, in all likelihood do better at home, I couldn't care for her full time at home because my husband and I both needed to work to pay the mortgage and support our sons. I also had enough self-awareness to know that I lack the patience for full-time care. I am best suited to short stints of quality care. With the support and considerable help of my husband, we took Mum to our home on the weekends and were rewarded with a marked improvement in her mood and her cognitive performance during and after each visit. My husband and I chose to apply our energy to making her life as enjoyable as possible within the constraints of our own abilities and limits, financial and otherwise.

Providing care for a relative living with dementia can be a positive experience. In fact, it has been associated with psychological benefits and better physical health for the care partner. However, there is no denying the considerable evidence that, for many people, looking after a relative with dementia can negatively impact on health and can take its toll on family life and relationships.

The reality is that you will have both positive and negative experiences. This book aims to help you to tip the balance towards the positive. The care partner stories and the self-assessments in the next five chapters will give you important insights into how you're coping and whether you have enough support.

The sixth and final chapter in this section examines the factors that help to make caregiving a rewarding experience with positive health benefits. Each chapter also has practical tips to help you to minimise the negative impacts of caregiving and maximise the positive aspects to benefit you and the person you care for.

CHAPTER 1

Burden

AUDREY AND MAY

Audrey, who cares for her 87-year-old mum, May, says: 'I've lived close to Mum and Dad since I got married really. They were fantastic when my children were small, helping with the childminding while I worked. Mum and Dad were a very self-sufficient couple and once my children were grown, I kept in touch with them almost daily on the phone and we regularly saw each other socially, for Sunday lunches, shopping trips to town, that kind of thing. But that all changed when Dad died suddenly five years ago. Mum became very depressed and dependent on me. She rang me constantly and expected me to drop everything to listen to her, run errands for her or visit with her.

'I hadn't realised how much Dad did for her and the more time I spent with Mum, the more I realised that things weren't quite right. Her condition got progressively worse and she was diagnosed with dementia three years ago. I am her sole carer. Mum and Dad did so much for me over the years, I really owe it to Mum to care for her now that she needs me. But I'm finding it really stressful. I am the only one of their four children who lives in the same country as Mum and so the role of carer was thrust upon me. I feel that I had no choice in the matter.

'I am really struggling to balance my job and my own family with caring for Mum. I love my job and am good at it but I'm not a natural at dementia caregiving. I feel like a failure. I'm not sure what I should or shouldn't be doing. My siblings all have strong and sometimes differing opinions. My two brothers, both senior execs

> in large multinationals, send me instructions and lists of things to do and expect me to update them regularly. My sister, Kate, in New York, is a complete mess – she just cries about the fact that Mum has dementia and tries to block it all out because she says it makes her too stressed.
>
> 'I am at the end of my tether. I'm tired all the time, I can't sleep, and I seem to catch every cold that's going. I find myself crying a lot and I can't see any light at the end of the tunnel unless I put Mum into a nursing home. She made me promise never to do this, but she is getting worse. It's risky leaving her alone. She really needs full-time care. I've already reduced the hours that I work but I can't give up completely as I have to pay my mortgage and support my children through college. Just thinking about putting her into care makes me feel ill, stressed and guilty.'

If, like Audrey, you are feeling overwhelmed, the tips at the end of each chapter may help you to find a better balance between caregiving and caring for yourself. Obviously, things like financial challenges will still be there, but the tips may help to alleviate some of the other stresses and strains that you are experiencing. This, in turn, may make you feel better able to cope with the situation, think more clearly and find solutions or support. Alternatively, the suggestions and advice may help you come to terms with the fact that you need professional help to care for your relative. Supplementing your care activities with professional in-home care services can be a sensible and life-changing choice, if you have the means to pay for a carer with dementia-specific training. If possible, explore the options early in your dementia journey; this will enable you to plan in advance and allow time, for example, for a needs assessment for state home-care or residential services or to explore what paid professional services would best suit your needs and how much they cost. Of course, not everyone has the option to plan ahead and some care partners reach a tipping point and have to make decisions around needing full-time residential care without any advance input from their relative.

Feelings

If you were to take part in research or visit a medical professional, they would describe the physical, psychological, social, emotional and financial challenges you face while looking after your relative as 'caregiver burden'. As you might expect, the term 'burden' refers to the work associated with caregiving, but importantly it also refers to the emotional and psychological toll that caregiving can take on you.

The level of stress that you experience as a care partner is related to how you view your current situation, your confidence in your own ability to cope and whether you think you possess the resources needed to carry out dementia caregiving. It also depends on whether you feel that becoming a care partner is something you chose to do or something you felt obliged to do. Care partners like Audrey, who feel trapped by their role and have negative beliefs about their own coping ability, experience more depression, have higher rates of illness and tend to move their relatives into institutional care sooner than those who don't feel trapped.

Guilt

Audrey feels guilty just thinking about putting her mum into care, to the extent that she feels physically ill and stressed at the prospect of doing something her mum might not want. Guilt is an unpleasant and powerful emotion, and I felt it often throughout my own caring journey. Guilt about not visiting Mum if I had to work late or guilt about not being home to cook the children's dinner because I was visiting Mum. Guilt about cancelling arrangements, guilt about not keeping up with friends. It seemed that whatever I did, whatever choice, I made, I would feel guilty about something or someone.

Our emotions play a key role in driving our actions, steering us toward things that improve our well-being or keep us safe. I find it helpful to think of emotions and feelings as pleasant or unpleasant rather than good or bad. Specific emotions and feelings nudge us toward specific kinds of actions. For example, hunger motivates us to eat because we want to get rid of the unpleasant feeling of hunger.[1] The pleasure we derive from eating tasty food motivates us to seek out and consume food again. Both the unpleasant feeling of hunger and the pleasure of taste associated with eating serve a function – they help to ensure that we eat, thereby enhancing our survival and overall quality of life.

Guilt, like hunger, is unpleasant – we want to make it go away. When we engage in acts of kindness, the pleasure centres in our brain are activated, motivating us to be kind again. The neurotransmitters serotonin and oxytocin – which make us feel good and support bonding respectively – are also released when we do kind things. The functional purpose of hunger is to make us eat so that we stay alive. The functional purpose of guilt is more complex, involving the interplay between our needs as an individual, societal norms and the demands of living in social groups. Guilt acts like an internal regulator, reminding us of what is expected and nudging us to act in ways that are acceptable within our social, cultural or family group, enhancing our survival and the survival of the group over generations.

Studies have shown that guilt prompts us to engage in actions such as apologising or making amends, which helps maintain social bonds. This idea is supported by findings that individuals who experience guilt are more likely to engage in behaviours that benefit the group, such as cooperation and altruism. It is possible that in early human societies, individuals who felt guilt after harming others or breaking social norms were more likely to repair relationships and maintain their standing in the group. This increased their chances of survival and reproductive success, leaving many of us with an inherited tendency towards guilt. In essence, feelings of guilt encourage us to engage in pro-social behaviours. The specifics of those behaviours vary across different cultures and contexts.

When we feel guilty, parts of the brain that help us judge our own actions and worry about what others might think or how they might react are activated. This is why Audrey feels so guilty about contemplating doing something her mother specifically made her

---

[1] This is what happens in a brain free from injury and disease. However, these signals may be disrupted in someone with dementia or a brain injury.

promise not to do. Guilt deeply influences the decisions we make, propelling us towards certain actions. While on the one hand it serves us well, guiding us towards behaviours that are aligned with social and personal expectations, it is important to remember that our drive to dissipate feelings of guilt can cloud our judgement and lead us to make unrealistic commitments. This is particularly true when caring for a relative with dementia. I know for sure that if I had acted on every feeling of guilt I had related to caring for my mum, my health, my job and my relationships with my husband and children would have suffered. My feelings of guilt towards Mum would have been replaced with feelings of guilt about my own family or my job. I found it very helpful to view the guilt I felt in my role as care partner as a starting point. Rather than acting solely to stop feeling guilty, I took a step back and looked at the situation in a more objective, rational way, taking account of my own limitations and my other roles and commitments.

Try to notice when guilt is pushing you to make unrealistic commitments. Take a step back, breathe, acknowledge your limits. Consciously consider all the factors that influence what you can or can't do. Guilt can make it really difficult to be objective; if this is the case, ask the advice of someone you trust to have your interests at heart to help you make an objective assessment and an informed decision. If you still struggle to take on board the rational justification for your choices, even if others lay them out for you, writing a 'for/against' list may help you to manage those powerful feelings of guilt. This is very important because higher levels of guilt are associated with increased symptoms of depression, anxiety and emotional distress among dementia care partners. The chronic stress of caregiving compounded by guilt can really take its toll. Unlike hunger, it is not imperative that you take the action that guilt propels you towards.

Guilt-tripping

Guilt-tripping, where care partners are made to feel undue guilt or responsibility for their actions or decisions regarding care, has been identified as a significant issue in caregiving scenarios, including those involving older people or chronically ill individuals.

Guilt-tripping in care partners often arises from multiple sources, including family members, friends, healthcare professionals and societal expectations. The effect of guilt-tripping on care partners is profound, leading to increased stress, anxiety and depression. It can exacerbate feelings of being overwhelmed and can negatively impact the care partner's ability to provide effective care. Long-term effects might include burnout and a decrease in overall life satisfaction. Your family, including your relative with dementia, can use guilt as a tool to manipulate you into doing what they want.

The truth of the matter is that, consciously or unconsciously, most of us have harnessed the power of guilt-tripping, to get our own way, to get someone to do something for us or even to elicit sympathy. A one-off guilt trip is unlikely to have serious implications for a relationship or for the well-being of the individual being guilt-tripped, but repeated exposure can have significant negative impact on both. The experience of guilt for the person on the receiving end can be accompanied by feelings of anxiety, sadness and regret and can cause muscle tension and disrupt sleep. Repeated exposure to guilt-tripping can contribute to the development or worsening of depression, anxiety and insomnia. To help you avoid such negative consequences, you will find practical advice on how to identify and manage guilty feelings and guilt-tripping later in this chapter.

Workload

It seems logical to assume that the burden you feel will relate directly to the amount of work you do as a care partner. But that is not the case. Some people who take on a considerable care workload experience no increase in their levels of stress, while others, like Audrey's sister, Kate, can feel overwhelmed by the revelation that their relative has dementia even if they don't actually do any of the caregiving.

People who feel they have the ability, the knowledge and the personal resources to carry out the caregiving role, and don't feel threatened by it, tend not to experience increased stress as a consequence of their caregiving responsibilities and workload. This book gives you the knowledge and resources to support you to develop dementia-specific caregiving skills. It will also help you to shift your perspective on caregiving to minimise stress, protect your health and improve the entire experience for both you and your relative.

PETER AND MARGARET

Peter, a former GP, is cared for by his wife, Margaret, who says: 'I feel like I am constantly walking on eggshells. Peter was a brilliant GP. In addition to working long hours, he volunteered on a number of committees and enjoyed playing bridge. We had a lovely and loving relationship. Peter was the perfect gentleman, a gentle soul and a great conversationalist. His dementia symptoms came on suddenly and I think he feels very ashamed and embarrassed because he won't leave the house anymore and won't have visitors.

'His dementia makes him highly anxious and quite paranoid. He follows me around the house constantly, asking me where I am going and what I am doing. His manner has become very gruff and authoritarian. He questions everything that I do. It takes all of my energy not to scream at him to leave me alone. I know it's the disease, I do, but I am not used to having him speak to me that way. I feel like I can't breathe having him follow me around all the time.

'I used to run my own small business and Peter used to take great pride in telling people that I once won Community Business Woman of the Year. I was well known locally and had a busy social life before the dementia but that's all stopped now because Peter won't let me out of his sight, let alone out of the house. I feel like I am losing myself.

'Some days he can get aggressive, which, I hate to say, really frightens me. It feels like there is a stranger living in the house, living inside Peter's body. He has become unpredictable. I am constantly on edge, never knowing what will happen next. Peter was a dependable, calm person who never raised his voice. I feel that I

> can't leave him with anyone else because he could lose control and I'd never forgive myself if he hurt someone.
>
> 'I'm 85 now myself and wouldn't be strong enough to fend Peter off if he lashed out. He hasn't yet, but sometimes I am afraid that he will. I would hate for that to happen, especially as the old Peter would never forgive himself if he hurt me. I miss Peter, I miss our conversations, and I miss being able to ask him for advice.'

There are many people like Margaret who are faced with behaviours that challenge every day. If Peter had open surgery, for example, rather than dementia, a community nurse would most likely be appointed to change dressings and monitor his wound. As healing progressed, the responsibility for changing his dressings might be passed on to his wife Margaret, who would be shown how to care for and dress the wound. In contrast, dementia is a very complex brain disease that gives rise to very complex, often challenging behaviours, yet for the most part dementia care partners, like Margaret, receive no community support and no post-diagnostic instruction or training. This book aims to fix that.

Behaviours that challenge

Some people living with dementia can, like Peter, behave out of character and become aggressive, agitated or disinhibited. Health professionals refer to these behaviours as neuropsychiatric symptoms or behavioural and psychological symptoms of dementia (BPSD). These symptoms can be much more disruptive and challenging for the care partner than memory loss. This may be because these behaviours can disrupt the emotional connection you have with your relative and can also make everyday activities like dressing, washing and eating more difficult. Not feeling safe or equipped to deal with these behaviours adds to stress.

Section 3 (page 181) takes an in-depth look at challenging behaviours with a view to helping you to understand, manage and minimise their incidence.

Assessment: Burden

Take some time to look at your personal situation. Completing the assessments in this section will help you to determine the level of burden that you currently experience. Often, our perceptions don't match our reality. Time can be distorted by how pleasurable or how difficult an activity is. Time goes faster when we are lost in the moment and time slows down when we find ourselves in difficult situations. For Audrey, her time at work, which she loves, goes by in a flash, while the time she spends caring for her mum, which she finds stressful, seems to crawl by. Completing the Care Activity Log on page 26 for a week will give you an accurate picture of your responsibilities as a care partner. Doing this will help you to identify where you need help and support and what activities you could delegate or even dispense with.

Time is one of the scarcest commodities for overburdened dementia care partners. When you read through the tips in this book, you may say: 'That's all very well and good. But where the hell am I going to find the time to do all that stuff when I barely have time to eat?' That is perfectly understandable, but remember that many of the tips a) can be tagged on to stuff you already do, and b) will actually give you a sense that you have more time, not less. Many of them just require a minute or two or a simple acknowledgement that being kind to yourself will make it easier to be kind to your relative.

I've lost count of how many diets I've tried over the years and the ones I've found most successful had just a few very clear simple rules. The least successful ones have involved keeping detailed records of the number of calories I consumed in every meal every day. I found it useful to record what I ate for the first day or two to give me a sense of how much I was eating and what foods were super high in calories. But after that initial learning period I just found recording everything I ate tedious, even when using a smart app. The purpose of keeping a log of what you do as a care partner is really a one-off exercise to give you an accurate picture of what you are spending your time doing. After that, the rules are simple: you need to create 'me time', you need to look after yourself and prioritise your health and well-being. Keeping the log will be tedious but it's an important exercise that will help you to decide whether you can combine activities, delegate activities or even eliminate activities altogether. It will also help you to identify the activities that a professional care provider could help with, and perhaps help you identify potential windows of opportunity for 'me time'. Try to remind yourself that self-care is essential, not optional. Book a slot in your calendar for self-care and see it as an appointment that you can't cancel. The key aim of this section of the book is to help you to achieve more balance between caregiving and looking after yourself. Completing the Care Activity Log is an important first step.

Start by logging the number of hours or portion of hours that you spend engaged in each activity each day. It doesn't have to be exact; your best estimate is fine. You don't want the log to become another burden! You will find examples of the types of activities that fall into each category in the Appendix on page 277.

Care Activity Log

On average, how many hours a week do you provide care? ____

Category	Day 1	Day 2	Day 3	Day 4	Day 5	Day 6	Day 7
1. Personal care for your relative							
Toileting							
Mobility							
Nutrition/Cooking etc.							
Support							
Medical							
Companionship							
Monitoring							
Appointments							
Other							
2. Household							
General housework							
Laundry							
Gardening							
Grocery shopping							
Banking/Finances							
Other							

Other							
3. Self-care							
Sleeping							
Eating							
Physical exercise							
Healthcare							
Socialising at home							
Socialising outside home							
Time outdoors							
Time in nature							
Reading							
Hobbies							
Other							

*If keeping this log for one week doesn't capture activities you engage in that take up considerable time but occur less than weekly, make a pro-rata estimate.

Level of burden

To determine your current level of burden, tick the box opposite each statement that best describes your current situation where:

- SA = Strongly Agree
- A = Agree
- D = Disagree
- SD = Strongly Disagree

Statement	SA	A	D	SD
1. I feel fresh and rested in the morning.				
2. My life satisfaction has suffered because of the care.				
3. I often feel physically exhausted.				
4. From time to time I wish I could 'run away' from the situation I am in.				
5. I miss being able to talk to others about the care.				
6. I have enough time for my own needs and interests.				
7. Sometimes I feel that the person I am caring for is using me.				
8. Away from the caring situation, I can switch off.				

9. It's easy for me providing the necessary nursing care (washing, feeding etc.).				
10. Sometimes I don't really feel like 'myself' as before.				
11. The care I give is acknowledged by others.				
12. Since I have been a care partner, my financial situation has decreased.				
13. I feel like I am being forced into this situation.				
14. The wishes of the person I am caring for are reasonable in my opinion.				
15. I feel I have a handle on the care situation.				
16. My health is affected by the care situation.				
17. I am still capable of feeling really joyful.				
18. I have had to give up future plans because of the care.				
19. It doesn't bother me if outsiders are aware of the sick person's situation.				
20. The care takes a lot of my own strength.				
21. I feel torn between the demands of my environment (e.g. family) and the demands of the care.				
22. I feel I have a good relationship with the person I am caring for.				
23. I have problems with other family members due to the care.				
24. I feel I should take a break.				
25. I am worried about my future because of the care I give.				
26. My relationships with other family members, friends and acquaintances are suffering as a result of the care				
27. I feel sad because of the fate of the person I am caring for.				
28. I can take care of other daily obligations to my satisfaction in addition to the caregiving.				

What your scores mean

Number of hours
- ☐ 1–7 hours per week = Low
- ☐ 8–23 hours per week = Medium
- ☐ 24–168 hours per week = High

For statements numbered:
1, 6, 8, 9, 11, 14, 15, 17, 19, 22 and 28, the rating is:
SA = 0, A = 1, D = 2, SD = 3

For statements numbered:
2, 3, 4, 5, 7, 10, 12, 13, 16, 18, 20, 21, 23, 24, 25, 26 and 27, the rating is reversed:
SA = 3, A = 2, D = 1, SD = 0

Calculate your total score by adding your score for each statement together.
My total burden score is ___

☐ 0–35: your burden is mild or non-existent.
You are not at risk of symptoms.
☐ 36–45: your burden is moderate.
You have an increased risk of developing symptoms.
☐ 46–84: your burden is severe or very severe.
You are at a very high risk of symptoms.

It is important to bear in mind that the above refers only to your care partner role. Like Audrey, you may also be holding down a job, looking after your own children or have other commitments, which could be either burdensome or beneficial.

If the number of hours that you provide care is medium or high and/or your burden score puts you at risk or at high risk, you will benefit from taking action to:

- Reduce the number of hours that you provide care.
- Reduce the level of caregiver burden that you experience.
- Create more opportunities for self-care.

Your Care Activity Log and your responses to the questions below, together with the practical tips on page 30, will help you find ways to reduce your feelings of burden and the time you spend actively caring, and to create more opportunities for self-care.

Many factors contribute to 'caregiver burden'. Your responses to the statements below, together with the information in your Care Activity Log, will help you to figure out the factors that influence your burden levels. Use your responses to the statements below to identify the factors that you need to address to reduce burden in order to gain more balance in your life. Tick all that apply.

1. ☐ I take on or do too much.
2. ☐ There are tasks that I could delegate to others.
3. ☐ There are tasks that are less important than my health and well-being and that of the person I care for.
4. ☐ There are times where I just need to be present in the house to supervise my relative when I am not engaged in any other specific activity.
5. ☐ I feel selfish and/or guilty if I put my own needs first.
6. ☐ I feel responsible for my relative's health.
7. ☐ I feel that if I don't do it, no one else will.
8. ☐ I feel that I am the only one who can do it properly.
9. ☐ My family place me in higher regard if I look after others than they would if I looked after myself.

Practical tips to ease your burden

Your answers to the questions above and your scores on the burden assessments, together with the information in your Care Activity Log, will help you to identify the practical tips that are most likely to ease your burden. Try to avoid the temptation to say 'I don't have the time'. Revisit your log and adjust it to free up some time.

When you are overburdened and stressed, it can be difficult to see things clearly. Consider asking someone else to look at your Care Activity Log with you. They may see opportunities for change more clearly than you do. Ask for help. If you still struggle to do this then it might be helpful to remind yourself that if you don't make adjustments to free up time for yourself, you will reach a point where you are no longer able to provide care due to your own ill health, burden or burnout.

Cognitive Behavioural Therapy (CBT)

Cognitive Behavioural Therapy (CBT) is a common psychological treatment that helps people deal with problems by changing how they think and act. The idea behind CBT is that our thoughts and perceptions influence our actions. The goal of CBT is to change unhelpful thought patterns and behaviours. It does this through two main approaches:

1. **Cognitive restructuring:** This involves challenging negative or inaccurate thoughts and replacing them with more balanced and realistic ones.
2. **Behavioural techniques:** These focus on how our actions and feelings influence each other. CBT uses practical methods like planning activities, learning new skills and problem-solving to help improve mental health.

CBT gives us tools to tackle a variety of mental health challenges and take better care of ourselves. Behavioural Activation is CBT speak for helping people start to engage in activities they enjoy or find meaningful because doing so can lift mood and reduce depression. For example, someone who has stopped doing hobbies because of depression might be encouraged to start with a small, enjoyable activity – a short walk or coffee with a friend, for example – and gradually add more activities over time.

In CBT, Activity Scheduling involves planning specific activities at set times to create a more structured day. This technique is often helpful for managing depression by setting up daily routines, like a walk, reading or a hobby, which increases the chances of having positive experiences.

Skills Training, another CBT technique, focuses on building social, communication and coping skills. For example, Skills Training to handle anxiety might include:

- Learning about anxiety and why it happens.
- Practising relaxation techniques to manage physical symptoms.
- Challenging unhelpful thoughts and replacing them with more realistic, positive ones.
- Practising skills in a safe setting (for example, through role-playing or 'acting as if') to build confidence.
- Applying these skills in real-life situations to develop a personalised plan for managing anxiety.

Problem-Solving involves learning a step-by-step approach to handling challenges. This might include identifying the problem, brainstorming possible solutions, choosing the best one and then testing it out. These skills can help you handle stress and challenges more effectively in your caregiving journey.

Set boundaries and limits

Setting boundaries and limits can be challenging, but it's worth trying to find a balance between your role as a care partner and the rest of your life. It's important to recognise that being a care partner is a significant part of your life and who you are. However, it's equally important to remind yourself that you are entitled to have a life of your own and relationships outside of caregiving. It's easy to fall into the trap of feeling that your life is somehow less important and must be put on hold to meet your caring responsibilities. It's not easy but the key is to give yourself permission to have a life of your own, have other relationships and meet the responsibilities and reap the benefits of those other relationships.

It's OK to acknowledge that you're not just a care partner, you are many other things too – whether that's a mother, spouse, friend, employee, artist or nature lover. Finding time for yourself and for those other roles may not always feel easy, but it's essential for your well-being.

If possible, try to delegate some caregiving duties or let go of tasks that aren't absolutely necessary. It might feel difficult at first, but accepting your own limitations can be empowering. Recognising both your limits and the incredibly important role you play as a care partner may help you realise that you can't do it all alone – and that's OK.

Allow yourself to rest, take breaks when you can, and know that by doing so, you are taking care of both yourself and the person you care for.

Protect 'me time'

Protecting a little time for yourself each day can be challenging, but it's worth aiming for. Take a look at your Care Activity Log to see if you can carve out even one 30-minute block each day to do something you genuinely enjoy. This could be as simple as phoning a friend, reading, stretching, meditating, gardening or treating yourself to a small luxury like a hot bath or a mug of hot chocolate. Finding time for yourself isn't always easy, especially with the demands of caregiving, but even brief moments can help recharge you. Chapter 10 offers practical tips to manage challenging behaviours, like those Margaret encounters, which can make finding 'me time' feel more achievable.

Become a guilt-free zone

Guilt can weigh heavily on dementia care partners, often affecting sleep, mood and overall well-being. Learning to recognise and manage guilty feelings is important – not only for your health but also for your relative's care. As discussed earlier, guilt can be a helpful guide, but if it leaves you feeling anxious, overstretched or overwhelmed, it may be tipping into burden territory.

Cognitive-behavioural approaches aimed at reducing guilt in those caring for people with dementia have been shown to help ease the burden that guilt creates. These methods focus on changing the thought patterns and beliefs that lead to guilt. The aim is to encourage healthier emotional reactions and behaviours.

Typically, these interventions are structured and led by trained therapists, either one-on-one or in groups, and are adjusted over time to fit the changing needs of the care partner. While working with a therapist is ideal, it is not always possible – thankfully, there are some techniques you can try on your own.

For instance, **cognitive restructuring** can help you identify and challenge irrational or unhelpful thoughts that trigger guilt. If you often think 'I'm not doing enough' or 'I'm a bad carer', cognitive restructuring can help you replace these thoughts with more balanced ones. For example: 'No one can be a perfect carer' or 'I'm doing the best I can with the resources I have.'

COGNITIVE RESTRUCTURING: EXAMPLE 1

Situation: Feeling that I am not doing enough for Mum.

Thoughts: I'm selfish and shallow spending precious time in the hairdressers or out with friends when I should be sitting with Mum. I'm lazy, too – I should do more stimulating activities with her.

Feelings: Guilty, inadequate, stressed, selfish.

Evidence that supports the thought: Sometimes I feel too tired to engage Mum in activities and feel relieved when she nods off. One day last week I left early to go out with friends and the week before I spent an entire afternoon at the hairdressers getting my colour done.

Evidence that doesn't support the thought: I provide daily care, manage her medications, make her meals and ensure she is safe and comfortable. I attend regular doctor and hospital appointments with her.

Alternative/balanced thought: I am doing my best with the resources and energy I have. Caregiving is challenging, and it's OK to have limits. I'm human and there are limits to what I can do. It's also important for my health and well-being that I keep in contact with my friends and look after my own appearance. Imagine if I wasn't there. Look at the difference I make every day.

Outcome: I feel more accepting of my efforts and less stressed about my caregiving role.

COGNITIVE RESTRUCTING: EXAMPLE 2

Situation: Feeling guilty about being irritated by and critical of my wife in the months before her diagnosis.

Thoughts: I'm a terrible person, I feel so bad for losing my rag with her. I should have been more supportive. I didn't show any compassion whatsoever.

Feelings: Guilty, regretful, sad.

Evidence that supports the thought: I sometimes lost my temper and was critical of her behaviour.

Evidence that doesn't support the thought: I was unaware of her condition and the changes it was causing in her behaviour. Since her diagnosis, I have learned more about dementia and understand that her actions were not within her control.

Alternative/balanced thought: I acted based on the information I had at the time. Now, with better understanding, I can be more compassionate and supportive.

Outcome: I feel more forgiving of myself and understand that my actions were based on lack of knowledge, not lack of care.

Deep breathing, progressive muscle relaxation and guided imagery can also help care partners manage stress and anxiety that accompany guilt. You can find tutorials and guided sessions for these techniques online. Many websites and apps, like Calm, Headspace or YouTube, offer free resources, including step-by-step instructions or audio guides that you can follow at your own pace. These relaxation techniques can provide immediate relief from intense emotions, enabling you to approach situations more calmly and with greater clarity.

Don't be taken on a guilt trip

Guilt-tripping is most likely to occur in relationships with people with whom you have a close emotional connection. Family members, including your relative with dementia, can be culprits. It can be intentional or unintentional. Sometimes it can be very clear that you are being manipulated – other times less so. Watch out for the key signs (see box on page 36) that someone close to you is trying to guilt-trip you into doing more than your fair share of caring, agreeing to unreasonable demands or taking on too much.

SIGNS THAT YOU ARE BEING GUILT-TRIPPED

- They subject you to the silent treatment.
- They remind you of mistakes you have made in the past.
- Their comments suggest you haven't done as much work as them.
- They remind you of favours they did for you in the past.
- They act as if they are angry with you but say there is nothing wrong.
- Their body language, expressions or tone make clear that they disapprove of what you are doing or the level of care you provide.
- They make sarcastic comments about the care you provide.
- They suggest you owe them or remind you of everything they have done for you.

Here are some practical things you can do when you encounter a situation where someone is trying to guilt-trip you.

- Calmly tell them how you feel. Let them know that you see they are trying to guilt-trip you into doing what they want, doing more, etc. Suggest that guilt-tripping will sour your relationship and ask for more direct communication going forward.
- Depending on the request, you can reassure them that you are not ignoring them. Tell them you know it is important to them. Be empathetic, validate their feelings while also clearly stating yours.
- Set boundaries. Be clear about explaining your limits, what you can do and what you can't. Explain the consequences of being pushed beyond your limits. It is critical that you stick to your limits and enforce your boundaries.
- You are more likely to give in to guilt-tripping when you don't feel good about yourself. Make protecting your well-being a priority. Being kind to yourself, practising self-compassion, working on your self-confidence and more generally looking after yourself will help you to resist being guilt-tripped.

- If the person persists in trying to manipulate you with toxic feelings of guilt, consider reducing contact with them. In the interests of self-preservation, you may need to consider ending the relationship as they clearly do not have your best interests at heart. For a variety of reasons, this may not be a realistic option and won't be possible, for example, if your relative with dementia is the one doing the manipulating.

It will likely be a steep learning curve, but it is important for you and for your relative that you take time off without feeling guilty. Don't let what your relative with dementia or other family members might think or say prevent you from taking time away from caregiving. Don't waste your precious 'me time' by feeling guilty. Try to schedule regular breaks into your day, even if it's only for a couple of minutes at a time to take some deep breaths, go for a walk, do some stretching or even a bit of mad dancing to release tension and reset yourself.

Delegate

If finding time for yourself feels like an insurmountable challenge, it might help to start thinking about ways to delegate. Asking for and accepting help can be hard, but it's important to give yourself permission to lean on others. You can use your Care Activity Log to identify tasks where a little extra support could make a big difference.

Consider matching these tasks with friends or family members based on their strengths, availability and preferences. It's OK to ask directly for help with specific things, and being open about your needs may lead to support you didn't expect. You might be surprised by how much time this could free up for you.

Remember, it's OK to accept help when it's offered, and try not to hold on to disappointment if it isn't. Everyone has their own stresses, and we don't always know what others are going through.

When family members, such as siblings, live far away or even in another country, why not ask them to assume the caring role when they visit so that you can schedule a holiday or some time off for yourself?

If, like Audrey, you have more than one sibling, you could ask them to stagger their visits across the year so that you can get a number of blocks of time off. If family can't help in person because they live far afield or can't visit for whatever reason, why not ask them to contribute financially so that you can pay for professional support? Having a paid professional to help with tasks, if you can afford it, is a reassuring way to free up time for self-care.

> **CHOOSING PROFESSIONAL HOME-CARE SERVICES FOR A RELATIVE WITH DEMENTIA**
>
> When selecting in-home care services, it's essential to approach the decision with clear goals in mind. Your Care Activity Log will help you to identify what you most need help with. If possible, involve the person with dementia and other family members in the discussion. You may also need to consult with healthcare professionals if your relative has medical needs. Consider the following:
>
> 1. Start by identifying what kind of support your relative with dementia requires. Identify the support that you and other family members can provide and make a list of the support or services that you would like the professionals to provide. This could be help with daily activities, personal care such as bathing and dressing, companionship, cognitive stimulation social activities or lifts to medical or other appointments. You can consult with healthcare professionals to create a detailed, personalised list of needs. Support requirements and service needs will change over time so this is an ongoing activity rather than a one-off.
> 2. Ensure that the individual you employ to care for your relative or the home-care agency you engage has specific experience in dementia care. Ask about their training and familiarity with managing dementia-specific behaviours and meeting dementia-specific needs. It is important to clarify whether they will send the same person every time. Ask if you can have an informal interview with the proposed carer. This might not be possible and, to be

frank, in my experience there is a scarcity of people trained to care for someone with dementia and you may have no choice. Having said that, since this person will be coming into your relative's home and interacting with your relative in important and often personal ways, I think it is very important to ensure that you feel comfortable with them, that they will be a good fit for your relative and are qualified to deliver the support that you both need. Below are some questions you could ask.

a) Could you tell us about some of the most rewarding and challenging moments in your previous job?
b) Have you worked with individuals with dementia before? If so, could you share a bit about that experience?
c) In your view, what qualities make someone a compassionate carer?
d) What do you see as your biggest strengths, and are there any areas where you're working to improve?
e) How would you handle a situation where the person in your care refuses your help?
f) If the person in your care gets up during the night and wants to go for a walk outside, how would you approach keeping them safe?
g) Can you give an example of a time when your skills were particularly helpful?
h) How do your friends describe you?
i) What drew you to caregiving as a profession?

You might also consider asking more specific questions relevant to your relative.

a) Mum sometimes imagines that she smells smoke and becomes frightened. How would you reassure her?
b) Dad frequently tries to leave the house at night and gets upset if he can't. How would you help him settle down?
c) How would you respond if my husband shows no interest in food? What would you do to encourage him to eat?

    d) If my wife misplaced her wedding ring and accused you of taking it, how would you handle this?
3. Ask the professional carer for their police clearance certificate and also ask for and check out their references. If your relative has complex medical needs, you might want a person who is certified in basic medical tasks like CPR, first aid or medication management.
4. Customise to suit your needs. This is a key benefit of in-home care. You can arrange care for a few hours or 24/7, depending on your needs and resources. This flexibility allows you to adjust care as the condition and your capacity and circumstances change over time.
5. Spend time with the professional carer. Make sure they are clear about what you need them to do and how you would like them to interact with your relative, etc. It might be helpful to provide them with a manual of sorts, with key information in writing. If possible – and it may not be – consider arranging a trial period before making a long-term commitment. This allows you to observe how the professional carer engages with your relative and, importantly, how your relative responds to the professional and to the new arrangement. Regular communication with the agency, the professional carer and your relative are crucial and will help everyone to adjust care plans as the dementia progresses.

HELPING YOUR RELATIVE ACCEPT IN-HOME CARE

Years before my mum had a diagnosis of dementia, my suggestions that she get someone in to help with cleaning and managing the house were met with a mix of horror at the very idea that she would let some stranger into her house and indignation at the implication that her house wasn't clean. Track forward several years to her first hospitalisation with UTI-induced delirium, when she agreed to having some home help if it meant she could leave hospital and go home. Here are some tips on how to first introduce the idea of in-home care:

- **Start slowly:** If possible, ease your relative into the idea of someone to help and support them by starting with short visits and gradually increasing the time spent together. This will allow them to get accustomed to the new person.
- **Frame it positively:** Try explaining the situation as having extra help rather than implying they need care. For example, say something like, 'This is someone who can help us with things around the house,' which can make it feel less threatening. I know this can be really challenging, especially if your relative is anything like my mum, who was very stubborn, strong-willed and set in her ways. You could also frame it so that the help is for you rather than for your relative.
- **Maintain familiar routines:** Keeping routines as consistent as possible can help your relative feel more comfortable with the changes. Encourage the professional carer to do things in ways that are familiar to your relative.
- **Give control when possible:** Allow your relative to have a say in the process. Involve them in choosing which tasks the professional carer will help with. This can help them feel in control and less anxious while also preserving their sense of independence.

MOVING TO A RESIDENTIAL CARE HOME

Residential care may become necessary, particularly in the later stages of the disease. If the decision has been made to move your relative into a residential care home, you will find some tips below on how to approach the transition and what factors to consider.

- **Choosing a care home:** Look for facilities that offer memory care services specifically designed for people with dementia. These homes often have specialised staff and environments that are better suited to the needs of those with dementia.

- **Environment and design:** Dementia-friendly care homes often have simplified layouts, circular walking paths and sensory rooms to reduce agitation. It's important to visit potential care homes with your relative if possible and observe how the environment might impact your relative's well-being.
- **Safety measures:** Ensure the care home has a good balance between safety and freedom of choice.
- **Social interaction and activities:** A good care home should offer opportunities for social interaction and stimulating activities tailored to the cognitive level of its residents. This can help improve mood and slow cognitive decline.

Helping your relative adjust to residential care

- **Visit frequently at first:** Frequent visits, especially early on, can provide a sense of continuity and help with the adjustment. Familiar faces during the initial phase can reduce feelings of abandonment. Some care homes insist that you don't visit for the first couple of weeks, arguing that it makes it more difficult for the patient to settle. It seems unnecessarily cruel to me and I suspect the more likely reason is that visiting makes life more difficult for the staff.
- **Bring personal items:** Decorating their new living space with familiar objects from home, such as photographs, favourite bedding or mementoes, can create a comforting environment.
- **Be patient with the transition:** It is normal for there to be some resistance or anxiety initially. Giving your relative time to settle in and gently reinforcing the benefits of the move (such as safety or more social interaction) can ease the process.
- **Communicate with staff:** Stay in regular contact with the care staff to monitor how your relative is adjusting. They can also give insights into how to address behavioural issues that might arise in the new environment. While many care homes are staffed

> by dedicated, caring, professionals, it's important for you as a care partner to remain actively involved in your relative's care. Building a strong relationship with the staff and maintaining open communication can ensure that your relative's unique needs and preferences are always understood and prioritised. If your relative doesn't have an independent advocate then you or another family member or friend need to take on that role, especially if your relative can no longer advocate for themselves.

Calling on friends to help

You don't have to do it all. Next time someone from your social circle offers help, refer to your list and say, 'Well, actually, it would be great if you could sit with Dad while I take the car for its MOT on Thursday' or 'I know you're a fantastic cook – if I bought the ingredients, would you make and blend a batch of soup that I can freeze for Mum?' There are bound to be lots of activities that you could delegate, as well practical tasks such as housework.

It is likely that a good portion of your time is spent just being there with your relative to ensure their safety. Simple things could make a huge difference. For example, if your relative is immobile or can't be left alone, could you ask a neighbour to sit with them for 15 to 30 minutes? This could allow you to get outside in the daylight and reap the benefits of a brisk walk while knowing your relative is safe. Maybe someone in your family could collect the prescriptions and make up the weekly tablet blister pack. Perhaps a friend could pick up a few groceries for you while they do their own weekly shop; alternatively, you could offer to shop for them if they sat with your relative while you go to the supermarket. Maybe you could ask someone, including family who don't live nearby, to help with form-filling, finances or health insurance claims if these are things you struggle with or would like to offload.

Breaking jobs down into small, manageable tasks can make it easier for people to help. You can share your task list with family and friends and let them choose the task they would like to help with. Online shared calendars and forms like Google Sheets are great for this, as everybody gets to see what needs to be done and who is doing what. It may even act as a motivator to get them to do more. Make sure to ask people if it's OK to share the calendar with others.

Get help as soon as possible. Don't wait until you become overwhelmed and exhausted. If you feel uncomfortable asking for help for yourself, remember the help you are asking for will benefit your relative so you could reframe your request as something they could do for your mutual relative.

DELEGATING

Máire-Anne

'When I initially moved home (to Dublin from Toronto, where I had lived since 1989), I naively thought there would be a 'one-stop shop' for everything related to dementia – what supports were available for my dad and me, etc. Sadly, this is not the case. So, I thought, 'Right, I can do this on my own, I will be grand, how hard can it be to look after my gorgeous dad in his own home.' So, I went to any and every information session that mentioned dementia. I quickly found that there was lots of information out there. However, it was all the same information, with several groups overlapping and doing the same type of info sessions, advocacy work, etc. I also came to the realisation that I couldn't do this on my own, and I would have to accept help from friends of my dad's when they offered, or indeed from my own friends. My mum used to say 'It is easier to give than it is to take,' which is so very true... I felt I was letting Dad down to 'allow' a friend of his or mine to come to his home for a cup of coffee in the morning so that I could go to the supermarket for groceries, etc. In actual fact, Dad so enjoyed the change of company, and I came back from the shops with my purchases, delighted with my solo shopping. Another friend offered to come every Saturday afternoon to watch the races with my dad (which they both enjoyed immensely) and

> they even used to have a "penny" bet between themselves, adding to the fun. It meant I knew Dad was being "looked after" without him *feeling* he was being "looked after", and I had four hours to myself to do whatever I needed or wanted to do. His friend loved the fact that he felt needed and that he was doing something to help his friend, aka my dad.'

Share experiences

While not for everyone, joining a care partners' support network can be very beneficial. Some care partners find it helpful to be with people who understand what they are going through. Learning that you are not alone in the sense that others experience the same emotions as you can be comforting. Discussing your experiences may help you to cope with anger, frustration and feelings of hopelessness. Sharing your experiences with others will give you some perspective and you may even pick up some tips and techniques that others in the group have employed successfully. You might also experience a boost to your own well-being by supporting others and sharing your insights and solutions.

One word of warning: if you do attend a care partners' group, be wary of those with a negative outlook who are more interested in complaining than finding ways to make things better. There is nothing wrong with complaining – we all need a little rant now and then. Complaining can spark others to help you or share their experience and the solutions they found, but what you want to avoid is for the complaining to become the focus. Hopefully, a support group – and this book – will help you to find some strategies to get yourself into a more positive, proactive place.

CHAPTER 2

Health

> **THOMAS AND ELIZABETH**
>
> 'One of the things I find most difficult to deal with is having to take Elizabeth with me when I go to the doctor, which I seem to have to do a lot more than I did before Elizabeth was diagnosed two years ago. I can't predict how long it will take to get her ready because some days she is agreeable but other days she can be really stubborn and dig her heels in, either refusing to get dressed or refusing to come with me. I can't leave her alone as I am afraid that she could quite literally burn the house down. Often, this means that I arrive at the GPs either too early or too late for my appointment. The waiting room can be difficult as Elizabeth can become agitated or say embarrassing things about the other patients,' says 82-year-old Thomas, who is the primary carer for his 79-year-old unmarried sister Elizabeth who moved in with him after his wife, Beatrice, died three years ago.

There is considerable evidence that dementia caregiving leads to a number of negative health outcomes including anxiety, depression, physical illness, hospital admissions and even reduced life expectancy for the carer. Many dementia care partners find themselves, like Thomas, visiting their GP more often and are at increased risk for numerous health issues including arthritis, ulcers, anaemia, diabetes and cardiovascular problems. Like Audrey, who cares for her mum, May (chapter 1), they tend to have lower immunity and poor sleep patterns. They also take more prescription medications and are more likely to use smoking and alcohol to alleviate stress or as a coping mechanism. Audrey is likely one of the four out of ten dementia care partners who live with depression, a mental health issue that also impacts on physical health since lower levels of depression are associated with better physical health and higher levels of resilience in care partners. If you are experiencing any of these health issues, you really do need to invest in some self-care.

Understanding unhealthy caregiving

Most loving relationships are characterised by mutual caring whereby each person wants to protect and enhance the other's well-being. Care is an integral part of parent-child relationships, spousal/life partner relationships and close friendships. It occurs naturally when we bond and tends to come with strong emotional connections. When Margaret's GP husband, Peter, developed dementia (chapter 1), it came as no surprise to her that she would want to protect him and become his care partner. Isn't that what they vowed on their wedding day all those years ago when they said 'in sickness and in health'? As the disease progressed and Peter began behaving out of character, Margaret felt a raft of mixed emotions: she felt short-changed because he would never be able to care for her and she felt betrayed by his behaviour.

She no longer felt that Peter would protect her, she missed the 'old Peter' and felt the loss of his support; but changes in Peter's behaviour also changed the dynamics of their relationship. Even when you know that your relative's altered behaviour is a consequence of the disease rather than a conscious choice, it is very difficult not to feel hurt, let down or even betrayed on some level. It can feel as if the unspoken rules of respecting and caring for each other have been broken. Margaret found the transformation of their treasured relationship particularly challenging to cope with.

Their 'couple friendships' seemed to fade out with Peter's diagnosis. Margeret no longer felt part of a couple. She felt grief and she felt abandoned. She found the isolation that she felt one of the hardest challenges she had to deal with.

When someone you care about develops dementia, the relationship can shift, often in profound ways. This can happen gradually, as it did for Margaret with Peter, who began behaving differently after the onset of dementia. Caregiving roles can become unbalanced, leaving one partner feeling burdened, especially when they must manage more of the day-to-day tasks alone. While these changes can feel overwhelming, there are strategies to help make this journey smoother and more manageable, preserving parts of your relationship even as it evolves.

The emotional toll of these changes and conflict with your relative can be tough, bringing feelings of exhaustion, isolation and depression. It's not easy but many care partners find that, with the right support, they can find new ways to connect, communicate and cope.

If your ability to cope is feeling stretched, this can impact your overall well-being and the well-being of your relative. Remember, though, that taking even small steps – like getting a little extra support, taking regular breaks or reaching out to friends – can make a big difference. These small actions help protect both your health and your resilience, allowing you to provide better care in the long run.

The onset and progression of dementia can be stressful for everyone involved. Long-term stress affects sleep and health, but there are tools that can help mitigate this impact. Simple practices like mindful breathing, staying active and maintaining a support network have been shown to help care partners manage stress and stay healthier. It will feel difficult at times, but focusing on manageable goals can help you take positive steps to support both yourself and your relative.

As dementia progresses, you may encounter physical and cognitive challenges in your loved one, from mobility issues to memory loss and, sometimes, behaviours like agitation. These can feel very draining, but there are approaches and resources – such as understanding triggers for certain behaviours or setting up a safe and comfortable environment – discussed in section 3 that can reduce these stresses. While caring for someone with dementia is undeniably hard, small, consistent actions can help create moments of calm and connection, which are invaluable for both of you.

Sleep

You will find some practical advice around good sleep hygiene at the end of this chapter and section 3 offers tips on how to manage challenging behaviours that can occur during the day or at night and which may impact negatively on your sleep. But first I want to share with you why sleep is important and why it is worth prioritising.

Sleep disturbances are common for people with Alzheimer's disease and other types of dementia, with research showing that 60 to 70% of people with cognitive impairment or dementia have sleep disturbances. These sleep issues can include trouble falling asleep, waking up frequently at night, or feeling unusually sleepy during the day.

In dementia, sleep disruptions often happen because of changes in the brain's natural sleep–wake cycle, symptoms related to dementia, or side effects of certain medications. These sleep problems don't just affect the person with dementia – they can also be challenging for you as a care partner, adding extra stress and making it harder to rest.

To help manage these issues, many care partners find that things such as keeping a regular sleep schedule and making the bedroom comfortable can be helpful. In some cases, doctors may also suggest medications, but this is usually done under close medical supervision.

The section that follows delves into why sleep is so important, and also highlights the negative impact that poor-quality sleep and insufficient sleep can have on your health – it doesn't make for joyful reading and my aim is not to depress but to help you to understand that prioritising your own sleep is of critical importance for your health and your ability to provide care for your relative.

You probably already know that getting around eight hours of sleep each night is one of the best things you can do for your health. Quality sleep plays a major role in how you feel, how well you function during the day, and in protecting your overall health. Even though this can feel hard to achieve, especially as a care partner, there are ways to improve both the quantity and quality of your sleep, which will have a powerful impact on your well-being.

Try asking yourself: how many hours of uninterrupted sleep do you usually get each night? If it's less than six or seven hours, it's normal to feel tired, but it can also affect your immune system, leaving you more open to infections. Research has shown that chronic sleep loss can also raise the risk of conditions like heart disease, stroke and Alzheimer's disease. It can also take a toll on mood, increasing the likelihood of anxiety or feeling down.

It's a lot to take in, and I don't want to add to your worries! The good news is that even small improvements in sleep can lead to noticeable benefits. Care partners often have more disrupted sleep and feel its effects during the day, so finding ways to protect your sleep – even if it's through short naps or improving sleep quality – can make a big difference. And remember, prioritising sleep isn't selfish: it's essential to help you stay resilient, both for yourself and for the person you're caring for.

Insufficient sleep messes with the hormones that control your appetite, so you end up with an amplified 'I'm hungry' signal and a reduced 'I'm full' signal. Have you ever noticed that when you are sleep-deprived, you don't just feel tired – you feel hungry too, and find yourself raiding the biscuit tin or snacking on crisps throughout the day. Research shows that even if you manage to get five or six hours' sleep at night, you are at risk of eating an extra 300 or more calories than you would after sufficient sleep. Sleep deprivation also makes it more likely that you will crave sweets, salty food and heavy carbs. I've been there and I know it's not easy to resist those cravings. With inadequate sleep we have less control, our drive to eat specific foods for pleasure increases and it is tougher for us to resist junk food. This kind of eating leads to an increased risk of obesity and type 2 diabetes, which in turn lead to increased risk of developing dementia.

I know when I gain weight, my first instinct is to look at my eating habits. In an effort to lose weight, I will try to restrict my calorie intake or eliminate the fatty and sugary foods that I have allowed unconsciously to creep into my diet. Like a lot of people, I will struggle to do this because it requires considerable self-control, which can be particularly hard in times of stress and when my sleep is disrupted. I have found that my personal experience supports what the science says – if I prioritise my sleep, the cravings dissipate and I find it easier to be more conscious and more disciplined with my eating. I seem to want to eat more healthily. With good sleep, I also find it easier to manage the stress in my life. Prioritising sleep will help you to regain control over your appetite and make it easier for you to maintain a healthy diet and manage the stresses of caring.

The reasons for care partner sleep disruption are complex and not yet fully understood. You might expect that being awakened during the night by the person with dementia would be the biggest contributing factor to poor sleep, but the research is inconclusive in that regard. The advice and suggestions in sections 2 and 3 should help to improve your relative's sleep, as will the suggestions at the end of this chapter, but my main aim is for you to consider adopting some of the practical tips in this section to improve your own sleep. Research shows that your sleep, as a care partner, may be disrupted by your own behaviour. Do you sacrifice time asleep to get some time alone or to catch up on chores or other work while your relative sleeps? I know this is a habit I developed when my children were babies and I learned the hard way through exhaustion and ill health that, in the grand scheme of things, having a spotlessly clean house is nowhere near as important as catching up on your own sleep whenever you can. Do you have an irregular sleep schedule? Do you eat late at night? Do you smoke or drink alcohol? Do you drink fluids close to bedtime? Do you do your worrying as you lie in bed at night? Do you scroll on your phone in bed? If you answer yes to any or all of these questions, you are not alone. These are habits that are easy to fall into, but breaking them and replacing them with healthier sleep habits is possible and will make a dramatic difference not just to the quality of your sleep but also to the overall quality of your life.

When it comes to sleep, your gender matters. Women, in general, are more likely to experience trouble sleeping at night than men. Women also experience greater excessive daytime sleepiness than men. Women are more likely to be care partners than men. Women are more likely to develop dementia than men. When care partners who are predisposed to sleep disorders – mainly women – are repeatedly awoken by their relative, they can develop habits that disrupt their sleep further. For example, they might drink caffeinated drinks to stay awake or nap for too long or too late, thereby disrupting their later sleep. There is a higher rate of depressive disorders among women in the general population and research indicates that depression in the care partner is also associated with poor sleep. This, of course, does not mean that men cannot be affected, it simply means that on average women are more likely to be affected.

You might be surprised to learn that care partners who do not live with their relative also experience poorer sleep than non-carers. Rather than being woken at night by their relative, they tend to lose sleep because of excessive worry and stress and because they can't switch off their thoughts about caregiving and so end up unable to enter sleep.

When it comes to sleep loss, stress is one of the main culprits. Brain chemicals connected with deep sleep are the same ones that tell the body to stop producing stress hormones. It's a vicious cycle, as insufficient sleep boosts stress hormones. Instead of shutting down, your body keeps pumping stress hormones, keeping you alert and awake. It doesn't take long for exhaustion and fatigue to set in. You become irritable, you will likely experience brain fog, making it hard to focus and problem-solve, impacting on your quality of life, work, relationships and your ability to care. All of which lead to more stress, less sleep and so the cycle continues.

The degree to which stress impacts on sleep is not the same for everyone. 'Sleep reactivity' refers to the degree to which your sleep is disrupted when you are exposed to stress. People with high sleep reactivity experience a drastic deterioration of sleep when stressed. Others can sleep like a baby despite everything going on. A family history of insomnia and being female increase the likelihood that you will have high sleep reactivity, which in turn is linked to increased risk of insomnia, a sleep disorder with strong links to stress, anxiety and depression. Insomnia affects more women than men and more older people than younger people. If you experience sleep difficulty three times a week for at least three months, it might be worth speaking to your GP, who will try to find out what's causing your insomnia so that you can get the right treatment. You might, for example, be referred to a therapist. Due to their side effects, doctors are unlikely to prescribe sleeping pills to treat insomnia, although if other treatments have failed and your insomnia is very bad, your doctor may prescribe sleeping pills for a limited period.

Insomnia might last for a short time, stick around for a while or come and go. You might have trouble getting to sleep or find yourself waking frequently throughout the night. For sleep to be restorative, you need to get seven to nine hours' sleep a night and cycle through five stages of sleep, each lasting approximately 90 minutes. This means that someone regularly getting ten hours' sleep but waking multiple times during the night may miss some of the stages and will likely experience symptoms of brain fog.

Assessment: Health

Please complete the following:

1. My general health at the present time is

Excellent ☐ Very good ☐ Good ☐ Fair ☐ Poor ☐

2. My overall sense of well-being at the present time is

Poor ☐ Fair ☐ Good ☐ Very good ☐ Excellent ☐

Centre for Epidemiological Studies – Depression (CES-D) Scale

Scale items
Below is a list of some ways you may have felt or behaved. Please indicate how often you have felt this way during the last week by checking the appropriate space. Please only provide one answer to each question.

	During the past week:	**Rarely** or none of the time (less than 1 day)	**Some** or a little of the time (1–2 days)	**Occasionally** or a moderate amount of time (3–4 days)	**Most** or all of the time (5–7 days)
1.	I was bothered by things that usually don't bother me.				
2.	I did not feel like eating; my appetite was poor.				
3.	I felt that I could not shake off the blues even with help from my family or friends.				
4.	I felt I was just as good as other people.				
5.	I had trouble keeping my mind on what I was doing.				
6.	I felt depressed.				
7.	I felt that everything I did was an effort.				
8.	I felt hopeful about the future.				
9.	I thought my life had been a failure.				
10.	I felt fearful.				
11.	My sleep was restless.				
12.	I was happy.				
13.	I talked less than usual.				
14.	I felt lonely.				
15.	People were unfriendly.				
16.	I enjoyed life.				
17.	I had crying spells.				
18.	I felt sad.				
19.	I felt that people disliked me.				
20.	I could not get going.				

Scoring:	**Rarely** (Less than 1 day)	**Some** (1–2 days)	**Occasionally** (3–4 days)	**Most** (5–7 days)
Questions 4, 8, 12, and 16	3	2	1	0
All other questions	0	1	2	3

The score is the sum of the 20 questions. Possible range is 0–60. If more than four questions are missing answers, do not score the CES-D questionnaire. A score of 16 points or more is considered depressed.

Add all items together to get your total score ___

Scores of 16 or more are considered to reflect high depressive symptoms. It is important to reiterate that this questionnaire is not a diagnostic tool, but it will give you insights into your depression levels.

What you can do

If you rated your general health and sense of well-being as fair or poor, it would be wise to take some steps to boost your health. Prioritising your well-being now can help you avoid health issues down the line and keep you feeling strong and resilient.

If your depression assessment score was 16 or higher, reaching out to a health professional would be beneficial. They can provide support and guidance tailored to what you're going through. But remember, if you're feeling concerned about your mood or mental health at any level, it's always a good idea to talk to someone sooner rather than later. Taking that first step can make a world of difference, and help is there when you need it.

Your responses to the following may help you to identify the steps you need to take to alter your habits, behaviours and thought patterns to improve your health.

1. ☐ I eat a healthy balanced diet.
2. ☐ I get sufficient sleep.
3. ☐ My sleep is of good quality.
4. ☐ My sleep is undisturbed.
5. ☐ I look after my health.
6. ☐ This is a new pattern of behaviour that has coincided with caregiving.
7. ☐ I have always put caring for others before my own healthcare needs.
8. ☐ I didn't look after my health even before I became a care partner.
9. ☐ I exercise for at least 30 minutes five times a week.
10. ☐ I eat regularly.

Practical tips for health

Your body likes routine and needs internal balance to maintain health. Stress can disrupt this balance in a way that can have serious consequences for your health. To help maintain this balance, you need to try to eat and exercise regularly. You also need to go to bed and get up at the same time each day, including weekends, to allow your body time to rest and recuperate after stressful events.

Prioritise sleep

Try to think of sleep as the most important thing you do every day. The specifics of how you make sleep a priority in your life as a care partner will depend on the nature and quality of your relative's sleep, your living arrangements and the nature of your relationship. Do you live together? Do you share a bed? Do you share responsibility for night-time care by taking turns staying over? Do you have access to a dementia-trained home-care assistant? The kind of supports available to you will depend on the funding, resources and training levels where you live. It's often a postcode lottery, which is neither ideal nor equitable. Regardless of the level and quality of support available to you, I hope that the general advice I provide in this chapter will help you protect your sleep, which you can adapt to your own personal situation. You will also find some information that might help you if you are a cohabiting couple or a family member or friend who shares their home with someone living with dementia or who stays over occasionally. Try to implement the sleep-promoting advice even if you only stay over once a week or once a month, and always when you are not on a caregiving sleepover.

Ideally, you should aim to get seven to nine hours' sleep each night if you are under the age of 65. If you are 65 or over, aim for seven to eight hours' sleep. If you cohabit or stay over a couple of nights a week, consider staggering bedtimes whereby your relative goes to sleep before you. This will leave you with some time each evening to develop a proper wind-down routine before bed. Or if you have begun staying over once or twice a week to support your relative, it may give you time to catch up with your own family or friends without disruption while you are away from home.

Creating a calming bedtime ritual can really help prepare you for a good night's sleep. Consider doing something relaxing, like taking a warm bath, meditating or listening to soothing music. When you soak in a warm bath, your body temperature rises. But as you step out of the bath and the water evaporates from your skin, your body starts to cool down. This cooling process helps signal to your brain that it's time to sleep, as our bodies naturally cool down when preparing for sleep. Lowering your core temperature after the bath makes you feel relaxed and ready for bed. This gentle drop in temperature helps you enter sleep more easily, as a cooler body temperature is ideal for falling and staying asleep. Try to resist the temptation to use this time to catch up on chores – you deserve a moment to unwind. Switching your brain to 'relax mode' before bed can improve your sleep quality and make it less likely that worries will wake you during the night.

If it's hard to prioritise time for yourself, remember that getting good-quality sleep will help you feel better equipped to handle the demands of caregiving. Your relative may still wake you during the night but at least you can minimise the number of times that your own stressful thoughts disturb your sleep.

If your relative takes a nap during the day and you live together or this is your designated day to care for your relative, you might consider taking forty winks also. Napping is a great way to repay any sleep debt that has built up. The timing and duration of your nap are critical to restorative napping. Don't nap after 3 p.m. – any later than that and you risk disrupting your night-time sleep. When it comes to duration, nap for less than 15 minutes or for at least 90 minutes. This is because it takes about 15 minutes to enter deep sleep and about 90 minutes to complete a full sleep cycle. Anything in between and you will wake up feeling groggy because you will be pulling yourself out of deep sleep. Set an alarm to manage your naps. Don't underestimate the power of a 15-minute nap – it can really perk you up and improve your alertness, with little or no grogginess.

Sleeping choices for couples

There is growing research on the effects of bed-sharing versus sleeping separately, especially in caregiving contexts. This is a complex issue where cultural and societal expectations can unduly influence personal choices without consideration of specific contexts and personal needs. Try not to let what is socially acceptable overly influence what, at the end of the day, is a very personal choice that can hugely impact not just the quality of your sleep but also your physical, mental and emotional well-being. There are benefits and drawbacks that will vary depending on your individual circumstances. Do try to make a choice that matches your personal situation and needs. There is no right or wrong choice. Choose what works best for you – and remember, this may change over time.

In western society, we tend to view sharing a bed as a barometer of the health of a relationship, but this generalisation fails to acknowledge important nuances. Yes, bed-sharing can be beneficial, but there are specific contexts and other factors that can make bed-sharing detrimental to the health of a relationship and the health of the individuals in the relationship.

It is true that sharing a bed can support emotional intimacy. Research suggests that bed-sharing also enhances sleep quality. In the general population, the sleep cycles of couples that share a bed become synchronised. In romantic relationships, a synced sleep pattern can offer several psychological and physiological benefits. Couples who tend to fall asleep together and wake up at the same time may wake up in a more positive mood and be less irritable, fostering healthier communication. When couples' sleep stages are aligned, both partners will go through restorative sleep at similar times, making them less likely to disturb each other's deep sleep, leading to a more restful night for both and reducing the likelihood of sleep-related conflict. In the general population, synchronised sleep can result in better mood, fewer arguments and an overall improvement in the quality of the relationship. For couples with conflicting sleep habits or where one partner snores, sleeping in separate beds or separate rooms can be beneficial, leading to improved sleep and even better relationship satisfaction.

Sharing a bed with a loved one who has dementia can be challenging, especially if your sleep is frequently disturbed during the night by your relative's needs. In caregiving situations, the dynamic shifts slightly. Your sleep quality can be compromised if your spouse experiences sleep disruptions as a consequence of their dementia. Separate sleeping arrangements may offer better rest for you, allowing you to maintain your health and emotional well-being.

Light

Managing your exposure to light over the course of the day can really improve the quality of sleep for both of you. Make sure you get exposure to natural light for at least 30 to 60 minutes every day. You can combine this with other healthy activities such as going for a walk, gardening or socialising with friends.

Try to get exposure to natural morning light as soon as possible after waking. For example, you could take a stroll in your garden or – weather permitting – sit outside for breakfast. Even if it's cold, you can don a hat and coat and grab a dose of fresh air and natural light while you have some tea and toast. If you live in a part of the world where the mornings are dark, expose yourself to bright light as soon as you wake up: for example, white light from a bedside lamp, not the blue light emitted from your phone and other devices.

If getting outdoors is problematic due to caregiving responsibilities or mobility issues, consider bright-light therapy with a special lamp. Research has shown that bright-light therapy improves sleep in people with Alzheimer's disease. Anything that improves your relative's sleep will minimise sleep disruption for you.

If possible, make the room you sleep in a technology-free zone; avoid watching television and using devices that emit blue light (such as laptops, tablets, smartphones) for an hour before bed. Make sure the room is as dark as possible at night. Avoid brushing your teeth under a bright light directly before you get into bed – the bright light will wake up your brain. Ensure that you both have a safe route to the bathroom should you wake during the night. If practical, avoid switching on ultra-bright lights. Cheap and cheerful low-level plug-in night lights can guide the way. A bedside torch and dimmer switches can all help.

Hydrate

Drinking lots of water is a great way to look after health, especially as we get older. Staying well hydrated can improve your cognitive functioning, stabilise your emotions and minimise feelings of anxiety. Water is essential for healthy digestion. Staying hydrated can help to keep your bowel movements regular and minimise bloating, flatulence and heartburn. If you allow yourself to become dehydrated, blood circulation can slow down, affecting the flow of oxygen to your brain. When you are dehydrated, your heart has to work harder to pump oxygen around your body, which in turn can make you feel tired and sluggish and impair your ability to focus.

Drinking plenty of water can boost your metabolism and help you to maintain a healthy weight because it can help you to feel full. Staying well hydrated can also minimise aches and pains by keeping your joints well lubricated, creating a cushion between the bones. Most of us don't drink enough fluids. As we age we are 20 to 30% more likely to become dehydrated. If you are over 60, you are at greater risk of dehydration. As we age, our sensation of thirst weakens. We may drink less than our body needs to stay hydrated because we don't feel thirst as quickly or intensely as we do when we are younger. As we age, our kidneys become less efficient at conserving water and it is easier to lose fluids from our body. In later years, we have a lower reserve of water: this means that we can dehydrate.

Drinking eight glasses of water a day is a good rule of thumb but the amount of fluid you need to drink to stay hydrated depends on many factors, including your activity level, your height, your body composition, your age and your gender, with men having slightly higher hydration needs. You can calculate how much water you should drink by dividing your weight in kilos by 30. For example, if you weigh 60 kilos, you need to drink 2 litres of water a day. If you prefer to use pounds rather than kilos then you need about half your body weight in pounds in ounces. For example, if you weigh 160 pounds you need to consume 80 fluid ounces of water a day, which is about four pints of water. Your intake needs will increase with physical activity so as a rule of thumb add 12 ounces of water for every 30 minutes of exercise.

Ideal fluid intake refers to all fluids, not just water. This includes beverages such as tea, coffee, milk, juice and even soups. Foods with a high water content, such as fruits and vegetables, also contribute to your daily fluid intake. The goal is to ensure your body gets enough fluids from various sources to stay hydrated and function properly.

Drinking most of your fluids during the day and restricting intake in the two to four hours before bed should minimise sleep disruption from waking to pee. Taking a nap during the day can allow fluids to be absorbed into the bloodstream. If you are prone to fluid build-up in your legs, elevating them will help to redistribute the fluids back into your bloodstream, reducing the need to visit the bathroom. Compression socks can help too. When you rest, nap or sleep the metabolic activity in your body is reduced. Your heart rate slows, your circulatory system calms, blood flow is more evenly distributed throughout your body, allowing fluids to be more efficiently absorbed into the blood stream. In addition, gravity exerts less influence on bodily fluids when you lie down for a nap. For example, fluid in the space between cells is more readily moved into the circulatory or lymphatic systems, which can promote better reabsorption into the bloodstream. When you sleep or nap you enter 'rest and digest' mode where various restorative processes, including the effective redistribution of water and electrolytes throughout the body kick in.

Healthy diet, healthy weight

I wish that eating a healthy diet and maintaining a healthy weight was as easy as writing about it. I know exactly what to do. Some days I do the right thing but most days I don't and that's why I am currently carrying excess weight, which I know is not only bad for my health but also affects my mood. Why is it so hard to follow such simple instructions? I know that the Mediterranean diet – rich in fruits, vegetables, whole grains and healthy fats – is a smart choice for getting the nutrients I need to support lasting health.

I really enjoy eating healthy soups packed with veg and salads full of fruit and nuts and seeds. Why, then, do I totally ignore my own advice more times than I follow it? Well, it's down to the fact that I am human. While we humans have an amazing ability to act rationally and make deliberate choices that are aligned with our goals, we are also driven by impulse and a strong desire for immediate gratification. On the surface, knowing we should eat healthily and maintain an optimal weight seems straightforward – just stick to nutritious foods and avoid impulsive choices. Sounds simple, but it's not, and when we are stressed and sleep-deprived it is even more difficult to resist our impulses. Reflective behaviour requires conscious effort – and it's hard work. In contrast, impulsive behaviour is effortless, unconscious, and is not only easy but provides immediate gratification. When I'm feeling stressed or overstretched, even though I know I could pull together a simple, nutritious meal, I'll grab a packet of crisps and a few chocolate biscuits and work through lunch.

To resist these impulses, it can help to plan ahead: keep healthy snacks like nuts, pre-cut veggies, or a batch of homemade soup on hand for moments when willpower runs low. Of course, not having crisps and chocolate in the cupboard would make life a lot easier, but that's easier said than done. Creating a routine, such as setting aside a few minutes each night to prepare for the next day's meals, can make it easier to stick to those considered choices rather than succumbing to unconscious impulse. And remember to be kind to yourself: resisting impulses is hard work, don't beat yourself up if you succumb. It's not easy, but small changes and preparations can make it more manageable. Remember, each time you choose a long-term benefit over a short-term craving or impulse, you're strengthening connections in your brain that will make it more likely you will make the healthy choice next time.

Rather than viewing blips along the way as failures, adopt the 80:20 rule. Aim to make healthy choices about 80 per cent of the time; when you do this, you give yourself the guilt-free flexibility for indulgences or less healthy options the other 20 per cent of the time. This approach promotes balance and sustainability, helping you to maintain healthy habits without feeling overly restricted or deprived.

For example, you might focus on eating nutritious meals, staying active and getting enough sleep most of the time (the 80 per cent), but also enjoy occasional treats, rest days or social outings without guilt (the 20 per cent). This mindset can make it easier to stick to healthy habits in the long run, as it avoids the all-or-nothing approach that often leads to burnout or giving up.

If you pack your freezer with frozen fruit and veg, you will always have something to eat in minutes. You can make a hearty, healthy soup in less than 15 minutes with an onion, a stock cube, boiling water and frozen veg. Salads are another great option. Toss a variety of salad vegetables and fruit in some olive oil mixed with lemon and garlic and sprinkle nuts and seeds on top. Or grill some chicken or fish and serve with steamed or roasted fresh or frozen veg. If cooking is not your thing, try to avoid overly processed food. Next time a friend asks if there is anything they can do to help, ask them if they could batch-cook some healthy meals for you or show you how to cook some simple Mediterranean food. With a bit of practice, you'll be able to whip up a tasty Mediterranean supper for two in the time it would take you to find the takeout menu.

In the later stages of dementia, Mum had trouble chewing and swallowing, putting her at risk for aspiration, which meant that she was likely to inhale food or fluids into her airways. Aspiration doesn't always cause complications, but it can lead to aspiration pneumonia.

If your relative has trouble swallowing, it's important to avoid dry foods or foods that require a lot of chewing and instead serve soups, smoothies and other moist meals using Mediterranean ingredients. Mum loved tomato soup – I think she liked the colour as much as the taste. If you need more personalised advice on what you or your relative should eat or how to attain and maintain a healthy weight, speak to your healthcare provider or speech and language therapist if one has been provided.

AISLING AND CARMEL

'Our speech and language therapist had great suggestions to promote and ease swallow and digestion for my mum, Carmel. She advocated the use of spices to stimulate taste centres. Doing this meant that Mum would continue with the meal rather than reject what she referred to as the "mush fit for a child". We'd often talk about her favourite foods, such as Indian curries, and modify those recipes for current use – she felt she had choice and autonomy over her "menu" rather than having to eat imposed "medical food".

'Mum was a great cook and passed that on to us children. We still enjoyed memory lane and cooked together while she could still "actively contribute". We kept up her annual traditions – for example, we made three-generation family recipe puddings in October and gave them as Christmas gifts.

'We exercised together too doing chair yoga and active retirement exercise classes. Siel Bleu[2] were great for combined carer/client classes, both in person and online. Also, we sometimes walked a friend's dog with them, lead attached to the wheelchair and then the little dog sat on Mum's lap on the way home if the dog was too tired!

'We made small incremental changes to our step count. For example, I used the upstairs bathroom during the day and when Mum's strength and general mobility declined she used the small portable step kit for legs and feet and put it on the table for arm and upper body exercises. We didn't need a gym or to change clothes or have a shower afterwards.

'I used to compile a "done/achieved" list at the end of the day as a gentle reward and recognition of my carer role. I still use that technique to this day.'

---

[2] Siel Blue is an international ogranisation that offers exercise programmes both online and in person, designed with a preventive approach to improve health through adapted physical activity, promoting autonomy and well-being to help individuals lead independent and fulfilling lives.

Exercise

Aisling and Carmel found ways to enjoy exercise together. It is important to find time to exercise. Scientists draw a distinction between physical activity and physical exercise. Being physically active includes any movements you make as you go about your daily life, such as vacuuming or helping your relative in and out of bed. Exercise is simply a type of physical activity that's organised, planned and repeated. Unlike everyday physical activity, exercise usually has a specific goal, such as improving strength, flexibility or overall fitness. Depending on the stage of the disease that your relative is at, you may find that your dementia caregiving role is physically demanding but leaves you with little time for more structured physical exercise.

Your Care Activity Log should hopefully have revealed some potential time slots that you could ring-fence for exercise. Depending on your relative's current abilities, you might even kill two birds with one stone by exercising together, like Aisling and her mum Carmel. Exercise is equally important for people living with dementia. The great news is that exercising every day will also improve sleep quality for both of you. Counter-intuitively, exercise will give you an energy boost and help you fight fatigue while also reducing tension and depression.

In addition, getting physically active will reduce your risk of more than 30 chronic diseases, including heart disease and dementia. There are 1,440 minutes in every day, so spend at least 30 of them doing some kind of physical exercise. If you can't initially carve out a continuous 30-minute slot for daily exercise, try breaking it down into manageable chunks – can you fit in three 10-minute sessions or six 5-minute bursts of exercises instead? I find it helpful to remind myself that some exercise is better than none, so even if I can only manage five minutes at a time, I know that's better than nothing – and as Aisling pointed out, doing exercise in short sessions means there's no need to change into exercise gear or have a shower afterwards.

However, it's not just about exercising for 30 minutes each day – you also need to change your sitting habits and move more throughout the day. If caregiving leaves you feeling exhausted, you may hanker after rest, but taking exercise throughout the day instead will give you much better payoffs in the health and energy stakes. If you can avoid sitting continuously for long spells and make a point of standing for a few minutes every hour, that's great. Encourage and support your relative to do the same.

How about getting the most out of any 'me time' that you manage to free up by combining exercise with socialising? Why not go for a brisk walk, for a swim, or to the gym or a dance class with friends instead of sitting down for lunch, coffee or drinks together?

Find aerobic activities you enjoy. Your caregiving responsibilities may mean that you will need to find imaginative ways to exercise or integrate physical exercise into your daily routine. Could you take a brisk walk together with your relative every day? Perhaps you could take an online exercise class at home while your relative takes a nap, or maybe they might join you. The internet is filled with online workouts that you can do at home. Dancing to music is a great option and vigorous housework and gardening count too. Attack them with gusto and see housework as a health booster rather than a chore. This is something I do myself and that simple switch in perspective really does make a difference.

Strength training and balance work are essential to guard against falls and frailty. Yoga, tai chi and Pilates classes will help boost your balance and workouts using only your own bodyweight are freely available online if you don't have access to free weights or a gym. Or you could ask for dumbbells for Christmas or your next birthday to help maximise your strength.

Enjoy yourself

Enjoyment is not frivolous – it is critical for your health and well-being and for that of your relative. It is a fundamental part of self-care. So please don't feel guilty about carving out time for enjoyment by delegating caregiving responsibilities. Things like dancing, drumming and juggling are fun and count as exercise. Dancing around the bedroom as you collect the laundry will boost your mood. You might feel a bit strange at first but anything that can give your mood a boost is worth trying. Why not practise juggling while your relative naps or watches TV? This might seem like a random suggestion, especially in the context of dementia caregiving, but the research shows that you will get a surge of dopamine, which will make you feel good as you rise to the challenge of learning to juggle. Learning to do other things will likely activate the same reward system: we feel good when we achieve something.

Prioritise your health

With everything else going on, it's all too easy to forget your own healthcare needs. You can't afford to put your health to one side while you prioritise the health of your relative. After all, you will be no good to anyone if you are unwell. Ask a relative, friend or neighbour to sit with your relative while you visit your GP so that you don't have the added stress of having to get your relative ready to go out with you. Follow your doctor's advice for managing any conditions that you have, don't skip your medications or hospital appointments, and keep your vaccinations up to date. If you are living with a chronic illness, get it 'flagged/on the agenda' early with your public health nurse, social worker, GP or healthcare agency. This can influence and even prioritise respite care allocation and care team support. Watch out for symptoms of depression such as crying more, sleeping more or less than you normally would, eating more or less than usual or a lack of interest in typical activities. I cannot stress often enough the importance of seeking professional help early.

CHAPTER 3

Stress

> **SARAH AND PATRICK**
>
> 'Even though I only care for Dad part-time, I feel like I am permanently stressed. My work is slipping. Last week I completely forgot to attend an important project meeting. My sister Ciara is great, we split the workload equally. Even so, I find it difficult to hold down a full-time job and keep on top of everything else. I visit Dad three or four nights a week and have him over for the day on Saturdays, which leaves little time to do my own housework and Dad's laundry. I'm exhausted and just can't think straight.'

This is how 42-year-old Sarah describes her life since her dad Patrick's diagnosis.

You don't need me to tell you this, but there is substantial evidence that assuming the role of care partner is stressful. In fact, caregiving fits the formula for chronic stress so well that it is frequently used as a model for studying the health effects of stress. Care partners with psychological illness and greater strain are at greater risk for poor physical health and illness. Caring for a person with dementia is more stressful and more damaging to health than caring for a person with a physical disability. Dementia care partners experience higher levels of stress and psychological distress and poorer physical health than other care partners and non-care partners. We'll first look at the indicators of stress before assessing how stressed you are. You'll then find stress-busting suggestions on page 81.

Brain fog

Sarah, who speaks about feeling exhausted and unable to 'think straight', may well be experiencing brain fog – a general term that describes a variety of symptoms, including mental fatigue and an inability to think clearly. If the following statements feel familiar, then you may be experiencing brain fog:

- 'I'm too tired to think.'
- 'I can't concentrate.'
- 'I just can't think straight.'
- 'I struggle to recall what I did yesterday.'
- 'I keep having to re-read the same sentence.'
- 'I can't work because I can't "tune out" other people's conversations.'
- 'My thinking is sluggish.'
- 'My life is like a game of charades, I can't find the right word, or I say the wrong word.'
- 'My language isn't as fluid or as rich as it ordinarily would be.'
- 'I've lost my sense of humour.'
- 'I'm struggling with small decisions like what to wear or what to have for dinner.'
- 'I keep bumping into things, spilling things, or slamming doors unintentionally.'

Brain fog affects people in different ways. It can be relatively mild or severe and can affect just one aspect of cognition or multiple aspects. In psychology, cognitive function is divided into domains. Each domain is responsible for specific functions.

The most commonly affected domains are complex attention, learning and memory, language, executive functions and perceptual-motor function. The speed at which you can process information slows and you may experience mental fatigue.

Most people will have experienced some, if not all, of these symptoms at some point in their lives. In fact, it is common to have these issues when you are sick with flu or other illnesses, if you have jet lag, or have been awake too long, have disrupted sleep, work long hours or are in a stressful situation. Brain fog is different to these short-term disruptions because it is persistent, occurs regularly and can interfere with the quality of your life, your relationships and your work.

Brain fog is not a disease or a disorder in and of itself, but it is real and can be incredibly debilitating. Chronic stress, insufficient sleep and poor nutrition in isolation or combined can cause brain fog. Add physical inactivity and low levels of mental stimulation into the mix and you have a recipe for brain fog.

Brain fog is also associated with some underlying health conditions (e.g. lupus, migraine, multiple sclerosis, Sjögrens, depression), medications (such as antidepressants, pain relief, anti-nausea, antihistamines) and hormonal changes (pregnancy, perimenopause, menopause). Speak to your doctor if you have other symptoms that may indicate an underlying medical condition, you suspect your symptoms are a side effect of medication or related to hormonal imbalance, or you notice that your brain fog has started suddenly or worsened significantly.

It's all too easy for dementia care partners experiencing brain fog to catastrophise and see their symptoms as signs of dementia. I want to make very clear that brain fog is not dementia. Please feel reassured that brain fog is generally temporary and can be improved and even eradicated by managing stress, prioritising sleep, taking regular exercise and eating a healthy diet even if you have an underlying health condition. Essentially, brain fog is a sign that you are not looking after yourself and a signal to take action to prioritise your health and well-being.

Assessment: Brain fog

Knowing your own symptoms will take you closer to positive change. A list of common symptoms of brain fog follows. Place a tick in the box next to any symptoms that you have experienced repeatedly or to the extent that it interfered with your everyday performance or quality of life over the last month. It is important that you only tick where there has been a change in your usual capabilities. We all differ in our abilities.

Some of us have always been a bit absent-minded or disorganised or have a short attention span. The key, in terms of brain fog, is whether you feel your performance or abilities have deteriorated from your usual baseline.

Executive function

1. ☐ I have difficulty making decisions.
2. ☐ I have difficulty solving problems.
3. ☐ I have difficulty making plans.
4. ☐ I am unusually disorganised or scattered.
5. ☐ I have difficulty multitasking.
6. ☐ I have difficulty thinking clearly, I feel foggy.
7. ☐ I feel confused.

If you answer yes to any of questions 1–7, your brain fog profile has an executive function component.

Attention

8. ☐ I have trouble concentrating.
9. ☐ I find it difficult to focus.
10. ☐ I have a short attention span.

If you answer yes to any of questions 8–10, your brain fog profile has an attentional component.

Processing speed

11. ☐ I experience slowed thinking.
12. ☐ I experience slowed learning.
13. ☐ I experience slowed processing of information.
14. ☐ I experience slowed reactions.
15. ☐ I am slow at completing routine activities.

If you answer yes to any of questions 11–15, your brain fog profile has a processing speed component.

Learning and memory

16. ☐ I have trouble with verbal memory (e.g. remembering a conversation).
17. ☐ I have trouble with visual memory (e.g. remembering an image).
18. ☐ I experience forgetfulness.
19. ☐ I have problems with short-term memory (e.g. recalling a limited amount of information such as a short shopping list after 10–30 seconds).
20. ☐ I have difficulty learning new skills.

If you answer yes to any of questions 16–20, your brain fog profile has a learning and memory component.

Language

21. ☐ I have problems expressing thoughts or understanding language.
22. ☐ I have difficulty finding the right word.

If you answer yes to question 21 or 22, your brain fog profile has a language component.

Visuospatial processing

23. ☐ I have problems navigating spaces (e.g. bumping into things)
24. ☐ I have problems recognising or drawing shapes.

If you answer yes to question 23 or 24, your brain fog profile has a visuospatial processing component.

Fatigue and irritability

25. ☐ I experience brain fatigue.
26. ☐ I feel mentally exhausted.
27. ☐ I experience irritability.

If you answer yes to any of questions 25–27, your brain fog profile has a fatigue component.

At the end of this chapter, you will find some practical tips on managing brain fog.

It's personal

As we saw with Audrey and her New York-based sister, Kate, the stress you experience because of caring will be different from the stress that another person will experience. This is because of differences in our resilience levels, circumstances, responses, resources and life experiences. Your age, gender, level of education, occupation and economic status, as well as the nature and quality of your relationship with your relative, will all contribute to how you respond. In addition to factors associated with your relative, such as their cognitive ability and the presence or absence of challenging behaviours, a host of other factors will influence the degree of stress that you experience as a care partner including: the size and quality of your social networks, access to caregiving training programmes, as well as your previous exposure to stressors and previous experience of caregiving.

You might expect that the number of activities you engage in to support your relative would dictate the amount of stress that you experience. But that is not the case – in fact, it is the resistance of the care recipient to help with activities of daily living such as washing, dressing and eating, rather than the activities themselves, that leads to stress in the care partner.

A sense of loss of a shared intimacy and engagement in previously shared activities – such as experienced by Margaret, who cares for her GP husband, Peter – are also stressors. While your relationship might change in terms of companionship, shared interests and support, it is important to remember that love, affection and warmth are all still possible. If you experience physical, emotional or mental exhaustion together with decreased motivation, poorer performance and negative attitudes towards yourself and others, it is likely that you are experiencing burnout and would benefit from visiting your GP.

Given the degenerative nature of dementia, many of the stressors you encounter will be lasting and will intensify as the disease progresses. Taking action to manage and minimise these stressors early on will help immensely. I hope you find the practical tips and tools peppered throughout this book helpful.

Roles

Other factors not directly associated with caregiving activities can be stressors too. For example, juggling your caregiving role with a job can also create conflicting pressures that lead to stress. It is helpful to acknowledge that your other roles, including those associated with work and family, are not necessarily detrimental. Switching perspective and reminding yourself that work and family commitments can be enjoyable and be positive sources of support and relief from the stresses and strains of caregiving can make a big difference to your stress levels. Having a social life and leisure time can also be beneficial; but unfortunately, caregiving obligations can limit opportunities to engage in social and recreational activities, leading to a sense of loss and stress. The tips later in this chapter will help you find ways to make more time for important restorative activities.

> **MILLY, WILLIAM AND KATHLEEN**
>
> 'I do most of the caring for Mum and Dad. I really don't think that the others realise what that involves or how much I actually have to do for our parents. I'm really fed up with my brothers and sisters giving their opinions on everything. It feels like they criticise everything I do. They want me to ask their permission first and expect me to do things their way. I try to be agreeable but to be honest it's getting ridiculous and at this point I feel like telling them that if I'm the one doing the caring then I get to decide how it's done. If they want to do things their way, well they're more than welcome to have a go,' says Milly about the constant emails, phone calls and WhatsApp messages from her older siblings on how she should care for their parents, William and Kathleen.

Family

Family conflict is relatively common when a family member has dementia. I know from personal experience that the equilibrium of family life may be disturbed, old grievances surface and new ones arise. If you are the primary care partner, you may encounter ongoing conflict with other family members. These conflicts often result from disagreements around the nature and severity of the disease and the most appropriate strategies for dealing with it, as well as the amount and quality of care and attention given by other family members to the relative with dementia.

Losing my 'self'

Caregiving for her husband, Peter, has prevented Margaret from engaging in activities and carrying out roles that she had previously enjoyed. This has led Margaret to feel a loss of her sense of identity and her sense of self. This is relatively common in care partners and the loss experienced can be further exacerbated by the fact that your life becomes increasingly intertwined with that of your relative. How you evaluate and describe yourself, including your psychological characteristics, your qualities and your skills, contributes to your sense of identity. What you think about yourself, your situation and your abilities matters.

Your self-esteem reflects the degree to which you view your qualities and characteristics as positive. A reasonably high degree of self-esteem is necessary for good mental health, while low self-esteem is associated with depressive symptoms. Audrey's sense of failure at dementia caregiving may well be contributing to her depressive symptoms. Many of the tips in this book are aimed at giving your self-esteem a boost. Feelings of captivity and the increasing demands of caregiving can erode positive perceptions of yourself and your sense of control over the forces that affect your life, leaving you vulnerable to stress.

Perceptions of stress

What you think and how you appraise a situation influences your body's stress response. For Margaret, characterising her days as unpredictable and believing that she was no longer in control of her life triggered anxiety and stress. For Milly, the criticism from her siblings was a constant source of stress. For Audrey, it was the sense that she had no support. Psychological distress refers to the extent to which you perceive that your current demands exceed your ability to cope. Sound familiar?

Assessment: Stress

Take some time to identify the specific sources of stress in your life – the triggers. Although there are commonalities across dementia care partners, stress triggers and responses are very individual and so it is important to identify what sparks the stress response for you. It may help you to keep a Stress Log for a few days.

Use the Stress Log template on page 76 to create your own version and log any stress you experience. If you don't experience any stress, leave the log blank. If you have more than one stress experience in any day, note down each one. This will help you to identify patterns.

- **Duration:** The total time from when you began feeling stressed to when you returned to feeling calm.
- **Stressor:** The thing, thought, person, situation, event, etc. that led to your feelings of stress – for example, email from family, your relative asking the same question for the umpteenth time, your children asking for help with their homework, having to ask your boss for time off for yet another hospital appointment for your relative.
- **Location:** Where you were – home, work, supermarket, etc.
- **Activity:** What you were doing at the time, for example, trying to dress your relative, trying to sleep, trying to think, working, etc.
- **Level:** Level your stress reached at its peak: 1 = mild, 2 = moderate, 3 = strong, 4 = severe.
- **Regularity:** Indicate the number of times you have felt stressed by this particular stressor in the past month.
- **Coping strategy:** Indicate any strategy you used to cope with the experience.

Stress Log template

Day	Time	Duration	Stressor	Location	Activity	Level	Regular	Coping strategy

Below is a series of statements that describe how you may have felt over the past week. Please read each statement carefully and indicate how much it applied to you by using the scale below.

Rating scale:
- 0 = Did not apply to me at all
- 1 = Applied to me to some degree, or some of the time
- 2 = Applied to me to a considerable degree, or a good part of the time
- 3 = Applied to me very much, or most of the time

Rate the following:

1. I found it hard to wind down.
2. I tended to over-react to situations.
3. I felt that I was using a lot of nervous energy.
4. I found myself getting agitated.
5. I found it difficult to relax.
6. I felt that I was intolerant of anything that kept me from getting on with what I was doing.
7. I felt that I was rather touchy.

Scoring

1. Add the scores for all 7 items to get the total raw score for the stress subscale.
2. Multiply the total raw score by **2**.

What your score means

Interpret your stress level based on the following ranges:

Normal: 0–14
Mild: 15–18
Moderate: 19–25
Severe: 26–33
Extremely Severe: 34+

What you can do

If your score indicates that you have high levels of perceived stress or is at the high end of moderate, then you need to take action to better manage stress, including seeking the advice of a health professional. The information in your Stress Log will help you to gain insight into the factors that trigger and influence stress levels. The log will also help you to distinguish between effective and ineffective coping strategies and which stress management tips might work best for you.

I am acutely aware that sole carers are particularly vulnerable to chronic stress and all of the things that brings. Bernadette shared with me her experience as the sole care partner for her late mother in the hope that it would encourage sole carers to take advantage of any and every support possible and prioritise their own health and their right to a life of their own.

BERNADETTE

'I was 33 years old when my mother was diagnosed with Alzheimer's disease and I became her full-time, sole care partner that year. I have no siblings. I have cousins and aunts and uncles, who distanced themselves completely from our situation from the beginning, and so I was a sole carer with no supports whatsoever.

'My mother's dementia changed her personality completely. She became paranoid, frightened, frustrated, anxious and had multiple challenging and responsive behaviours. After a hip fracture, she no longer knew who I was and was often violent towards me. We lived in total isolation. I could not leave the house and could not leave my mother unattended for even a short period of time.

'My mother refused to go to bed at night because she did not recognise our home and therefore told me every night that she was not going to go to bed in somebody else's home. So, we slept in chairs. For years. There was little sleep, no relaxation of any kind and stress increased all the time. I had no idea where to turn for help or what steps to take to manage my stress even a little.

'Dementia dismantled life as we knew it. I can't accurately describe the loneliness, despair, isolation and fear I experienced. Those years had long-term effects on both my mental and physical health. Stress completely overwhelmed me and I found that not only did it have a major effect on my health during the years I was caring for my mother, it resulted in long-term health problems that continue today.

'There was nobody to ring to talk to about what was happening because my friends back then were my age and so had no understanding of what I was going through. I was the only child of older parents. I despaired and in many ways I gave up on life. Alzheimer's had a brutal impact on our lives. But I also have a message of hope for sole carers. My mother was sick for 16 years. I was her sole carer for 8 years. It completely broke me. My mother died in 2017.

'I still struggle a lot with the aftermath of my carer's journey but I am slowly rebuilding my life. I had a superb GP who got me back on track slowly. I needed a lot of help and support after my journey caring for my mother ended. That is why I am so concerned for other sole carers.

STRESS MANAGEMENT FOR SOLE CARERS

Bernadette

'Make early contact with your local Alzheimer Society. Ask for their help and support. They are excellent and they truly understand the struggles and needs of sole carers.

'Work on the necessary legal things as early as possible. Power of Attorney[3] and Enduring Power of Attorney are so crucial. Sorting these things out as soon as possible following diagnosis will help avoid a lot of stress and worry later.

'Ask for a Public Health Nurse[4]. Public Health Nurses can be excellent support and excellent advocates.

'I started to write a daily journal. I didn't have anyone to talk to so it helped to write my thoughts in a journal. It was my way of

---

[3] Lasting Power of Attorney in the UK.
[4] Or District Health Nurse.

unloading the stresses and worries of the day, at the end of the day. I wrote very honestly. I wrote things like "I'm frightened," "I don't know what to do." It's not the same as talking to somebody but it is a way to acknowledge how you are feeling and to check in with yourself each day.

'There are many wonderful and free resources online now to help manage stress. Breathing techniques and gentle exercise that can be done at home and don't require any equipment are very effective to help manage stress. Apps like Headspace are also useful and effective.

'TV and radio frightened my mother as she thought people on TV were in our home. Radio caused her a lot of distress as she could hear the voices but could not understand where they were coming from. So I kept both radio and TV turned off. I had a small radio with headphones and I used that to listen to news and some music. This helped me a lot. I love music and sport and being able to enjoy them occasionally made a positive difference for me.

'Organisations like Aware[5] now provide excellent advice and online support for mental health problems like anxiety and depression. This can be done using email, text or online courses in stress management. I completed the online Aware course in mindfulness-based stress management earlier this year. It is an excellent programme consisting of one 2.5 hour meeting each week. It provides an excellent set of skills and techniques to manage stress.

'Recognise the signs of stress, depression and anxiety. Talk to your GP about them before they escalate and develop into bigger problems. Don't be afraid to contact helplines like the Samaritans. Sometimes just talking to a stranger for a few minutes can help so much. Aware also have an excellent helpline now. The Alzheimer Society[6] also provide an excellent and compassionate helpline.'

---

[5] Aware is a depression and support service in Ireland.
[6] The Alzheimer Society of Ireland – in the UK Alzheimer's Society.

Practical tips to manage stress

It is chronic, prolonged stress rather than caregiving per se that leads to health problems. Funnily enough, too little as well as too much stress has been shown not to be good for you. Following the practical tips below will help you to find your stress sweet spot.

Once you know your personal triggers, you need to establish whether the stressor can be changed or not. Many of the tips you will find in this book will help you to take action to change or eliminate some dementia-specific stressors. However, given the nature of the disease and your role, there will be many stressors that you cannot change. But this does not mean there is nothing you can do to reduce the associated stress. Changing how you respond to a stressor can be just as effective as eliminating the stressor altogether. Try out as many stress-reducing techniques as you can until you find the ones that work best for you.

Be present

Being 'in the moment' will also help you to stay away from negative thoughts or memories that can spark anxiety, stress and depression. Have you noticed yourself becoming more forgetful recently? Have you missed appointments, like Sarah, or do you find yourself frequently forgetting what you are doing midway through a task or halfway up the stairs? Absent-mindedness is a common sign of stress. When you are stressed, it can be difficult to keep focused on the task at hand. Being present and focused on what you are doing while you are doing it is a natural antidote to stress-induced absent-mindedness.

Rooting awareness in your body, such as feeling the soles of your feet connect with the ground while walking or focusing on breathing in and out, can tie you closer to the present moment and take your focus away from things that may be distressing you. When you are doing something with your relative – for example, helping them to dress, or applying moisturiser to their hands – try to be fully present in that activity. It is natural for your attention to wander, and you may find yourself distracted by distressing or depressing thoughts. Talking yourself through a task can keep you focused and present in the moment; so too can awakening your senses. For example, noticing the scent and texture of the hand cream, watching the motion of your hands and the way the cream spreads and dissolves can not only keep you grounded in the moment but also can make the experience more enjoyable and even more meaningful.

Being fully present when you interact with your relative, whether verbally or physically, can nurture a richer, more meaningful connection. It can open more subtle communication between you – the spoken word is just one way we express ourselves. When we actively listen and observe, it cultivates a deeper bond.

Yoga, meditation and tai chi are helpful ways to reduce stress and remain grounded in the present moment. If you can't make it to a class in person, there are lots of good ones to be found online.

Embrace routine

Human beings have a fantastic ability to carry out actions without consciously or actively thinking about them. You and I call these automatic actions 'habits'. It's been reported that more than 40 per cent of our actions each day are habits. This is an energy-efficient way for your brain to operate in the most routine circumstances.

Your brain loves routine. It constantly scans your behaviour, looking for patterns and routines to turn into habits. As much as we benefit from being present in the moment, we also need to be able to perform many tasks on autopilot. The conscious, thinking part of the brain uses up more energy than the unconscious part of the brain responsible for executing habits, which are an energy-efficient way of getting routine tasks done. Without habits, the human brain would become overwhelmed by all the choices and decisions about how to act and behave that need to be made through every minute of every day.

Turning chores into habits is a great way to relieve stress and brain fog and reduce feelings of overwhelm. Let's take laundry, for example. Does the overflowing linen basket in your bathroom make you feel stressed every time you go for a pee? Do you do it on a set day of the week or do you do it at random times when you have a free moment or when you run out of socks? If you were to follow through on a decision to make Monday laundry day, after a few weeks your brain would identify this as a routine suitable for automation. Once it becomes a habit, it will seem easier and less of a stressor. Go through your Care Activity Log and identify chores that you could turn into habits by doing them at a certain time every day or every week, depending on the tasks. Developing routines in this way can really free up headspace and energy for doing things that are fun or meaningful.

Healthy behaviours

Use healthy behaviours to manage stress. If stress is prolonged or chronic, it can trick you into narrowing focus to the extent that you fail to set aside time for yourself, for physical exercise and other leisure activities. This is particularly true for dementia caregiving, where it is easy to fall into the trap of focusing only on the disease and how it affects you and your relative.

Stress can lead to overeating and unhealthy food choices. In the short term, stress can suppress appetite, but in the longer term, if stress becomes chronic and is left unmanaged, cortisol, like lack of sleep, can increase your appetite and your motivation to eat. Stress can also make it difficult to fall asleep and stay asleep.

Regular exercise, a balanced diet and sufficient sleep are great ways to manage stress. Try not to rely on alcohol or drugs to reduce stress. Instead, follow the tips in this book and take practical steps to reduce stressors or change your response to them.

Laugh

Stress can steal your sense of humour. Ironically laughter is the ultimate stress buster and humour helps us all to cope with the unthinkable. Laughter actually reduces levels of the stress hormone cortisol. Remember, it is still OK to have a laugh and a good time. Dementia doesn't steal from your relative the desire to laugh and have fun, so have fun with them. I think I laughed more with my mum in the few years that she had dementia than I did in all of the other years put together.

Don't underestimate the power of humour and laughter: connect with a friend who makes you laugh, read a funny book, listen to a humorous podcast, watch a comedy or surf the internet for funny videos. Find ways to hold on to your sense of humour. Make a point of laughing at least once every day, especially if you don't feel like it. There are also laughter classes and laughter yoga – there is even a global belly laugh day on 24 January every year. You'll find classes online and you may even find some in your local area.

Laughter activates the immune response and so protects you against illness and infection. It can be therapeutic to spend time with others laughing and talking about things not related to caregiving, as well as talking about your fears, emotions and caregiving experiences. 'If I didn't laugh, I'd cry' is a phrase I use often when talking about stressful events or encounters. I find seeking out the funny side a great way to manage stress. With Mum, my husband and I made a conscious effort to focus on having fun with her in the moment rather than wallowing in tragic thoughts about dementia. When she did things out of character, like flirting with my husband, there was no embarrassment; he just played along, and she had fun and enjoyed the attention.

Be realistic

It's helpful to set realistic goals for yourself and recognise that sometimes 'good enough' really is better than perfect. Taking on too much can lead to burnout, so know your limits and aim for what's achievable rather than aiming for perfection. The same goes for those around you: avoid expecting too much from others, as it can lead to frustration and disappointment for everyone involved. Accept that others might not handle tasks exactly as you would, but letting go of control can be a healthier, more practical choice than trying to do everything on your own.

Clear the fog

Adopting healthy habits – including prioritising sleep, managing stress, exercising regularly and consuming a healthy, balanced diet – is the best way to eliminate brain fog in the longer term. In the shorter term, here are a couple of things you can do to manage symptoms while you work on developing healthier habits.

Avoid multitasking

When you attempt to do two things at once, you'll probably perform each task more slowly and make more mistakes. Far better, and less stressful, to do just one thing at a time. When you do something important and potentially dangerous like driving, or helping your relative to come down the stairs, give it your full attention. Essentially, multitasking is a myth and is more accurately described as task-switching because your attention is rapidly switching back and forth from one task to the other.

We all do it – we might chat with our relative while doing something else like cleaning the kitchen – and yes, we might save some time doing this, but we miss out on a genuine opportunity for improving the care experience for both of us. When interacting with your relative, try to focus solely on that if you can. You'll be surprised at how it will improve your connection and communication.

In addition to doing one activity at a time, try to finish things you start as much as possible. Unfinished tasks can add to feelings of stress. When you finish a task, you get a little buzz and will feel more energised and better able to take on the next task.

Remove distractions

Your eyes receive approximately 200 megabits of information flow every second. Your brain cannot process all the information from your senses. To make sense of the world around you and to avoid becoming overwhelmed, your brain filters out irrelevant information and filters in relevant information. You can assist your brain in this task by decluttering your surroundings, especially in places where you need to concentrate. Brain fog limits your ability to ignore distractors, so removing as many of them as possible from your environment will help you to focus and concentrate on the task at hand. Reduce noise, turn off the radio or TV or go somewhere quiet. If your relative likes the company of the background noise but you find it distracting or irritating, consider investing in noise-cancelling headphones so you can block out the noise if it is bothering you. Listening to soft calming music at a low volume on regular headphones can help to drown out distractors also. Remove visual distractors. For example, if you are trying to complete a complicated form, remove anything from your line of vision that might remind you that you have lots of other things to do, like the laundry or paying bills.

CHAPTER 4

Support

> **GLADYS AND MIKE**
>
> 'I haven't spoken to another soul in six days. It's tough to get out of the house with the icy footpaths and my bloody hearing is gone so bad now I can't use the phone because it's a bit pointless and if I'm honest more stressful than it's worth. I can't make out what anyone says on the phone, but I can hear their sighs of frustration when I ask them time and again to repeat what they said.
>
> 'I've always liked being useful and suffered terribly from empty nest syndrome when my children left home. I don't see looking after my husband, Mike, as a burden. I don't begrudge him a moment of my time. I'd even go so far as to say I enjoy looking after him. I just wish this damn dementia didn't rob him of words. I miss our chats so much.'

It's fantastic that Gladys, who is 87, hasn't lost sight of the fact that caring for someone with dementia can be rewarding and enriching, but equally important is the fact that she acknowledges that she feels isolated and lonely. Staying connected to close friends and family, who can provide much-needed social support, is vital. Finding ways around barriers to social connection, such as hearing loss or mobility challenges, is also essential. Technology can be a great help for someone like Gladys. With reduced hearing, seeing the person speaking on video call can make it easier to understand what they're saying. Speech-to-text technology, which turns spoken words into written text in real time, can also be beneficial. High-tech hearing aids and amplified telephones can make communication clearer. Features like a separate control to boost volume through the handset and compatibility with mobile phones and wireless devices could make a huge difference.

If you are not comfortable using technology, are not confident with computers or not familiar with technology, seeking support from a local community centre or library that offers computer literacy classes can be helpful. Additionally, you might consider asking a tech-savvy friend or family member for guidance on using new tools. Organisations that support care partners often have helplines or provide workshops to help navigate useful technology and other dementia-specific supports, making it easier for carers to stay connected and informed.

Social connection

Spending time with friends and being in social situations can be incredibly beneficial, helping you to feel more positive and less stressed. When you care for someone with dementia, it is all too easy to let the social side of your life slide. Maybe you are missing the chats you had with colleagues over coffee at work because you have cut down on the hours that you work. It's quite the challenge to find time to do everything. Time-saving choices like giving up your evening course or getting your shopping delivered might buy you more time but deprive you of important opportunities for social contact. Encourage friends and family to pop by for a chat. If the person with dementia is your partner or parent, you may feel, like Gladys, that you are losing an important confidant/e. Remember that you can still share memories or stories of your day with them or talk through any problems or decisions that you are grappling with – they may not respond as they did in the past, or they may surprise you with a moment of insight, but just saying things out loud may help if you are feeling lonely. Ensuring that your relative has as many opportunities as possible for social activity can also pay dividends for you in terms of meeting other care partners and simply enjoying events.

We don't usually think of socialising in the context of our physical health but loss of social connection is as bad for your health as smoking 15 cigarettes a day, being obese or being physical inactive. Feeling socially isolated can increase the risk of health issues like high blood pressure, depression and even dementia. Prioritising social connections, even in small ways, can make a big difference. Making time for a quick chat with a friend, scheduling a regular coffee meet-up or finding local care partner support groups can all help you stay connected and supported.

The quality of support you receive really matters. Positive, caring support – like a friend who truly listens or who offers to help – can lower your heart rate and blood pressure more effectively than neutral or negative social interactions. Maintaining a solid network of social support while being a care partner is not easy but it is particularly beneficial to your physical and mental well-being. Research shows that this is because the more challenging or upsetting a stressful situation is, the more you benefit from having a supportive network around you. When you have a support network you will cope better, feel less emotional distress, have good mental health, enhanced self-esteem and better heart health.

The amount of support that people perceive they have does not generally equate with the amount of support they actually receive. I know that sounds weird, but it highlights the fact that what you think matters. Surprisingly, the amount of support you see yourself as having is more strongly associated with health than the actual support you receive. When you *feel* regularly supported and socially integrated, your brain interprets these experiences as safety signals that change the processing of stressors in your brain and body. In simple terms, feeling supported by people who care about you makes a difference to your mental and physical health. When you manage to grab some free time, phone a good friend for a chat or make a firm date in your diary to go for a walk with your favourite cousin.

Perceived social support

Read each statement carefully. Indicate how you feel about each statement.

Circle 1 if you **Very Strongly Disagree**
Circle 2 if you **Strongly Disagree**

Circle 3 if you **Mildly Disagree**
Circle 4 if you are **Neutral**
Circle 5 if you **Mildly Agree**
Circle 6 if you **Strongly Agree**
Circle 7 if you **Very Strongly Agree**

		Very Strongly Disagree	Strongly Disagree	Mildly Disagree	Neutral	Mildly Agree	Strongly Agree	Very Strongly Agree
1.	There is a special person who is around when I am in need.	1	2	3	4	5	6	7
2.	There is a special person with whom I can share joys and sorrows.	1	2	3	4	5	6	7
3.	My family really tries to help me.	1	2	3	4	5	6	7
4.	I get the emotional help and support I need from my family.	1	2	3	4	5	6	7
5.	I have a special person who is a real source of comfort to me.	1	2	3	4	5	6	7
6.	My friends really try to help me.	1	2	3	4	5	6	7
7.	I can count on my friends when things go wrong.	1	2	3	4	5	6	7
8.	I can talk about my problems with my family.	1	2	3	4	5	6	7
9.	I have friends with whom I can share my joys and sorrows.	1	2	3	4	5	6	7
10.	There is a special person in my life who cares about my feelings.	1	2	3	4	5	6	7
11.	My family is willing to help me make decisions.	1	2	3	4	5	6	7
12.	I can talk about my problems with my friends.	1	2	3	4	5	6	7

Your score

This questionnaire measures your perception of social support from **family, friends,** and **significant others.**

To calculate your total score simply add up your scores for each of the 12 statements and divide by 12. Scores range from 1 to 7, with higher scores indicating greater perceived social support.

- **1.00–2.99:** Indicates a lack of strong social connections or support from one or more sources.

- ☐ **3.00–5.00:** Suggests an average level of perceived social support, which might indicate room for improvement in certain areas.
- ☐ **5.01–7.00:** Reflects a strong sense of social connection and availability of support from family, friends, and significant others.

You can also break down your scores to find out where you are well supported and who you might turn to for additional support.

Family support
Tot up your scores for statements 3, 4, 8 and 11 and divide by 4.

Friends support
Tot up your scores for statements 6, 7, 9, and 12 and divide by 4.

Significant other support
Tot up your scores for statements 1, 2, 5, 10 and divide by 4.

High scores on any of the three specific subscales (e.g. family support) suggest that you perceive strong support from that source. Low scores on a subscale may indicate an opportunity to enhance support from that particular group (e.g. strengthening relationships with friends).

What you can do

Your responses to the following questions may help you to decide what steps you need to take to boost your social support.

1. ☐ I have received offers of help but declined them.
2. ☐ I have help but it is not enough.
3. ☐ I have help but not with the things that I would like.
4. ☐ There are people whom I could ask to help.
5. ☐ I don't know how to ask for help.
6. ☐ I don't know what to ask for help with.
7. ☐ There are local services that I could make use of, such as respite or home help.
8. ☐ I could afford to pay someone to help.
9. ☐ I promised to always look after my parent/partner.

Practical tips to improve social support

Social support can be broadly divided into practical support and emotional support. Practical support refers to various types of help, including assistance with housework, transport and finances – booking a cleaner to come in once a week or asking someone you know to help with researching a good savings account. Emotional support is any action from a friendly chat to a positive text message, from hugs to hand-holding, that communicates care or concern and offers empathy, acceptance, reassurance or comfort. You will do best if you have a network that allows you to tap into both kinds of support.

Social support is not the same as being part of a support group. Support groups tend to be structured meetings of care partners led by a care partner or facilitator. In contrast, a social support network is an informal network, comprised of your friends, family, colleagues, neighbours and wider community, whom you can rely on for support in times of stress.

Stay connected

Sometimes, being sociable can seem like the last thing on earth you want to do when you feel exhausted. But it's important to resist the temptation to curl up in a ball and withdraw when you're stressed. It is very tempting to shut others out of your life because you need time alone to think (or not think!). You might also avoid others in order not to inflict your stress-induced crankiness or irritability on them. If you can, notice when you tend to do this and try to continue to reach out and communicate with others. Also try to avoid cancelling or rearranging plans when things are getting you down or you're particularly stressed. Remind yourself, if you can, that these are the times you'll benefit the most from some social interaction or a change of scene, and prioritise them.

Seek support from friends, family, befriending organisations and, if necessary, health professionals. If you have let friendships lapse because of the demands of caregiving, why not try reconnecting in person or via social media. Most people will understand why you let things lapse.

Saying hello to an old friend on Facebook or responding to an Instagram post if you're online can often start a conversation.

If your network has diminished for other reasons, try to make new friends at your support group or by taking part in community activities, or reach out to your neighbours. Could you carve out some time to join a Women's Institute or a Men's Shed? Could you volunteer on a local community committee? I know it might sound crazy to suggest volunteering when you might already feel overwhelmed but as the old saying goes 'a change is as good as a rest'. Volunteering provides a social outlet and being kind to others triggers the release of feel-good hormones in both the giver and receiver. Befriending services offer companionship to people who would like extra social contact through a weekly volunteer visit or telephone call. Befriending services are designed to alleviate the negative impacts loneliness has on mental and physical health. It can be tough to take that first step and admit that you are lonely. There is no shame in being lonely. If you feel lonely, it just means that you are human. The pain of loneliness is your brain's way of prompting you to get socially connected, just like hunger pangs prompt you to eat. I know that befriending volunteers get as much out of the service as the people that they visit. Most befriending services operate on a national basis with local branches and volunteers. Google 'befriending services' or ask your GP or health nurse for local contact details and take advantage of the services they offer.

How to ask for help

It can be daunting to reach out, so start with small steps. Share how you're feeling with a trusted friend or family member, even if it's just mentioning that you're overwhelmed or tired. This opens the door to further conversations about support.

When you do ask for help, being specific about your needs can make it easier for others to step in. For example, instead of saying 'I need help', you could say 'Could you come by for an hour so I can run errands?' or 'Would you mind preparing a meal once a week?'

Connecting with other carers via a support group can be a great way to learn how they ask for help and what works for them. Listening to their stories can inspire you to find the right words and confidence to reach out.

What to ask for help with

Identify key stress points: take note of what tasks or times of the day are most stressful for you. It could be handling evening routines, getting groceries, or simply needing some time for yourself. These moments are a good starting point for asking for support.

Review your typical day and list everything you do. Your log will help you to identify tasks that could be delegated, even if it's just for a short time. For example, help with housework, meal preparation, or taking your relative for a walk.

Think beyond physical tasks: emotional support is just as important. Ask a friend to come over for a cup of tea and chat, or request someone to join you for a social activity. Even watching a movie together with a bowl of popcorn could help you unwind.

Sometimes it helps to talk to a professional or an organisation: a social worker, a community health nurse or a volunteer at your local Alzheimer's Society, who can suggest practical areas where support would be most beneficial and help you build a network.

Practical examples of what you could ask for

- **Respite care:** This allows you to take a break while someone else takes over caregiving duties temporarily.
- **Help with errands:** Ask for help with grocery shopping, picking up prescriptions or other errands.
- **Transportation:** Ask for help getting your relative to appointments or social activities.
- **Home support:** Ask friends or family to help with cleaning, laundry or meal prep.
- **Companionship for your relative:** Having someone spend time with your relative while you take time to rest or do something for yourself.

Reaching out for help and knowing what to ask for may take time to feel natural, but remember, caregiving is not meant to be done alone. Accepting and seeking support can greatly improve your well-being and enhance your ability to care for your relative.

> **SHOW YOURSELF SOME LOVE**
>
> Practise self-compassion. As a dementia care partner, there's no doubt that you are well practised in showing compassion towards your relative. When is the last time, if ever, you afforded yourself the same level of compassion?
>
> To be truly self-compassionate, you need to combine social connection with self-kindness and non-judgemental, mindful awareness. This means treating yourself the same way a caring person would treat someone else, wanting to ease your own pain, staying balanced and not focusing too much on any one thing, and feeling a sense of connection with everyone else, sharing in the ups and downs of life. There's a wealth of research demonstrating the benefits of self-compassion for psychological well-being, including reduced anxiety and depression and improved happiness and life satisfaction. Self-compassion may have a soothing effect on our fear centres since it is associated with reduced activity in the amygdala, a part of the brain involved in fear and stress responses. Consider making a gentle commitment to show yourself some kindness and understanding. Try to be aware of your thoughts and emotions, letting them flow without judgement or harshness. Instead of getting caught up in every feeling, see if you can simply acknowledge them and let them pass. Sometimes, connecting with others can make a big difference too; reaching out, even in small ways, can help you feel supported and less alone. Being kind to yourself will take pratice but it is a valuable habit to nurture.

Give and receive

Supporting others is a powerful way to build and strengthen your social network, benefiting both you and those you help. When you actively participate in a network of support, you give and receive, creating a cycle of connection and mutual benefit. For example, staying in touch with friends or family through a quick call or message can brighten their day and give you a sense of belonging. Listening to someone share their challenges or celebrating their achievements shows you care, deepening your bond.

Expressing gratitude is also key. Letting people know how much you appreciate them creates a positive, supportive environment. And when someone you know is going through a tough time, offering to help in small ways or simply being there to talk can be uplifting for both of you.

You might think you're too drained to support others, but helping someone else can actually be energising. Focusing on someone else's needs, even briefly, can distract you from your own worries and leave you feeling more connected and fulfilled. Social support is a two-way street, and engaging actively in it can improve your well-being, reduce stress and foster a sense of community for everyone involved.

Choose wisely

Choose wisely who you spend time with. It is important to remember that your social network should help to reduce your stress, not increase it. You need support, not someone who will add to your stress. Try to be aware of situations and people who leave you feeling drained and be cautious around excessive negativity or criticism. It's also helpful to steer clear of those who may encourage behaviours that aren't supportive of your well-being, like overindulging in alcohol.

Family can be a wonderful source of support but for many care partners family members are a source of serious stress. If the latter is the case, you may need to take action to minimise contact in order to protect your own health. For example, if multiple WhatsApp messages from siblings about your relative are stressing you out, suggest creating a Family WhatsApp Group for urgent issues only and graciously mute the busy one that is a source of ongoing stress.

Human contact

Remember the importance of human contact and a hug. It can be hard to ask for help and even when we do, most of us are likely to ask for help with housework and care-related tasks. Of course, practical help is welcome, but you also need emotional support. Ask people to just be there, to visit you and be a listening ear for you. It can be hard to imagine yourself asking for help but it is well worth the effort. There are multiple ways you could approach this, so just choose the one that feels the least uncomfortable for you. You could be direct and say: 'I really need some company and a friendly ear. Could you come by just to chat for a bit? I'd love to catch up and have someone to talk to.' You could bring it up when someone comes to visit your relative: 'When you come to see Mum, it would be really nice if we could sit down together too. Sometimes I feel like I have lots of things going round my head, and it would be a relief to talk things through with someone who understands.' You could reach out to someone you trust and let them know you could do with some comforting: 'It's been a rough few days, and I realise I could really use a hug and some time to just unwind with someone. Are you free for a visit soon?' Rather than having to approach friends/family every time you need support, you could try asking for a regular check-in: 'Would you mind checking in on me once in a while? Sometimes I get so caught up in caregiving that I forget to take time for myself, and it helps to have a friend who reminds me to pause and chat.'

Don't be afraid to let your vulnerability show: 'It feels a bit awkward to ask, but I think I just need someone to be with me for a while. Not to help with chores – just to share some company. It makes such a difference to know someone's there.'

Lack of affectionate physical contact is associated with higher levels of stress hormones. But social contact, like giving someone a hug or holding their hand, can lower stress hormones and even lower blood pressure and reduce pain. This is great advice for caring for the person with dementia, but remember that you need human contact too – don't be afraid to reach out and ask for a hug.

Cultivate a confidant/e

For many care partners, their relative with dementia has always been their prime confidant/e. It's not easy to accept that as their dementia symptoms progress, this may no longer be the case; but it is important to acknowledge and worthwhile to nurture a relationship whereby someone you already trust now becomes that confidant/e. Having at least one close confidant/e can significantly enhance your quality of life compared to having none.

Dementia caregiving can be a rollercoaster of emotions. It is important that you have an outlet where you feel safe sharing your emotions and experiences. This confidant/e can be a friend or a relative that you trust, but it can also take the form of a support group where you can share, seek and exchange practical information with one another. Expressing yourself and sharing the challenges you face may lead you to solutions; but even if it doesn't, simply talking about your troubles can make you feel lighter, less burdened and less alone.

Use supports and services

Do some research on available supports in your local area. Your doctor, Citizens Advice or local Alzheimer's Society should also be able to put you in touch with local support groups and other services such as health teams and social workers, community meal services, day care, befriending and respite programmes. Consider paying for someone to help with housework and care if you are in a financial position to do so. If you have financial concerns as a consequence of caregiving, seek advice and take advantage of all the grants and supports that you can. Again, your local Citizens Advice, carers' associations or Alzheimer's Society should be able to point you in the right direction.

CHAPTER 5

Coping

SALLY AND ANDREW

Sally, whose widowed dad, Andrew, lives with her, says 'I'm very fortunate I can work from anywhere once I have Wi-Fi and a laptop. Most of the time Dad is very agreeable and easy to manage so I can combine work with caring. The only real problem I had was that Dad would act up, shouting, and banging his head with his hands every time I had to take a phone call, which really wasn't ideal especially if it was a work call. I found it very stressful to see Dad so agitated and distressed and since it could take a long time to calm him down afterwards, I knew I needed to do something. But I wasn't sure what I could do so I asked at the local care partners' support group. A few members in the group suggested that I keep a diary to see if I could identify any triggers or patterns.

'To be honest I didn't think there was much point in keeping the diary since I figured that it was pretty obvious that Dad's behaviour was a reaction to me paying attention to someone else on the phone. I remember my children doing something similar when they were small if I was yapping on the phone to friends for too long. Nonetheless I decided to keep the diary anyway since I felt I couldn't look for other solutions from the group without trying the diary first.

'For the most part the diary confirmed my theory that Dad only became agitated when I was on my phone. But keeping the diary helped me to notice that his agitated behaviour started before I started talking on the phone. Actually, it started as soon as my phone rang. I knew I was on to something when Dad became similarly agitated when a car alarm went off on the street. It seems that the pitch of my ringtone and the alarm were similar, and both triggered something in him that made him feel agitated. By the way he was banging his head I realised that the sound was excruciating for him.

'It was easy to find a relaxing ringtone that didn't bother Dad. He loves Schumann, so I chose Schumann's "Dreaming". Dad still gets agitated when a car or house alarm goes off but that's very rare. When visitors call, I ask them to put their phones on vibrate. It's amazing the difference that these small changes have made to Dad's life and to mine.'

Coping

Coping basically means how you react to or deal with stressful situations. Sally found a healthy and effective way to cope with a situation that she and her dad found stressful. There are various coping styles that people tend to use to handle stress and challenges. Research has established that some methods are effective and promote well-being, while others are less helpful and can even worsen stress over time. The problem-focused/solution-focused coping adopted by Sally is considered the healthiest and most effective coping mechanism.

Confronting problems directly and seeking solutions – known as problem-focused coping – is generally considered the healthiest and most effective way to cope with stressful situations. The aim of problem- or solution-focused coping is to solve the problem, eliminate it or decrease it. Problem-focused coping will usually involve defining the problem (for example, Andrew's bouts of agitation), seeking solutions (for example, his daughter, Sally, asking for suggestions at the support group), making choices (Sally keeping the diary even though she didn't have faith in its usefulness) and taking action (changing her ringtone and asking visitors to put their phones on vibrate). In essence, Sally adopted a problem-focused approach. She identified the problem, sought advice and followed the suggestion to monitor and record the situation; this in turn led her to a solution. She successfully managed the situation by tackling the problem directly. By removing the trigger, she essentially eliminated the problem, which benefited both herself and her dad, Andrew.

Managing your interpretation of the situation is another effective, active coping strategy. How we think about and perceive things influences how we react, how we behave, how we feel and how we cope. Changing our perspective, changing the meaning we give to a situation, can make all the difference in terms of whether we find the situation stressful or not as Jean's story illustrates.

JEAN AND ROBERT

Former schoolteacher Jean, who looks after her husband, Robert, admits: 'At first, to my shame, I treated Robert like a bold child when he wouldn't comply while I tried to dress him every morning. It was a horrible way to start the day, but I just felt like I was going backwards in time to when our children were small or when my students at school were being wilfully disobedient. Every morning was like a battlefield. On a carers' course, I learned that my bullying approach was part of the problem. It stung at first but not for long because it helped immensely to acknowledge that Robert is still my husband and recognise that he deserves to be treated like an adult.

'Robert still has difficulty dressing but once I changed my perspective from seeing him as a bold child to seeing my husband who needs my support to deal with the consequence of his brain malfunctioning, I became much more patient and allowed more time for dressing. After all, there was no reason to rush. Now if I feel stress and agitation rising, instead of tut-tutting and taking over control of dressing Robert I focus on my breath and on Robert's hands as he slowly dresses himself. I silently assist with the bits he can't manage. I gently encourage and guide while giving him the time that he needs to do as much himself as he can.

'I found that once I gave him time in silence without criticism, he could actually do much more himself than I had realised in my

> rush to get the job done. Instead of the stressful time that it once was, dressing has now become a pleasant ritual for Robert, and a meditation of sorts for me. We are a team focused only on the present. Robert leads the dressing dance and I am happy to follow.'

Jean recognised that her behaviour and her interpretation of the situation were causing great stress both to herself and to Robert. Rather than actively trying to change the situation, she chose instead to change how she interpreted it. By simply changing her perspective, she transformed what was a stressful daily occurrence into an enjoyable and meaningful encounter with Robert.

MARIA AND ELENA

Maria has been caring for her mother, Elena, who has mid-stage Alzheimer's disease. One of the most challenging aspects of Elena's condition is her 'sundowning', a behaviour associated with increased agitation and confusion that typically occurs in the late afternoon and evening. Sundowning is discussed in detail in section 3, and can involve difficult behaviours such as pacing, shouting and resisting care, which Maria finds extremely stressful.

One evening, as the sun began to set, Elena became increasingly restless. She started to pace around the house, opening and closing doors loudly and repeatedly asking Maria where her late husband was. Maria felt her own stress levels rising as she tried to calm her mother, fearing the night would be long and sleepless. Remembering the techniques she recently learned in a support group, Maria decided to focus on managing her own stress symptoms to remain calm and effective in caring for her mother. She started by taking deep, slow breaths to centre herself. Maria found this approach helpful, and she now practises mindfulness. She does this by consciously bringing herself to the present moment, acknowledging her feelings of stress but choosing to focus on her breathing and the immediate needs of the situation. Over time, Maria has noticed that her own calmness seems to soothe her mother's agitation. Maria now anticipates the sundowning and dims the lights, closes the curtains and puts on some calm music that Elena likes. She no longer tries to correct her mother's confusion about her late husband; instead, she calmly redirects the conversation to fond memories they share, showing old photos and telling stories from those times, which helps distract Elena. Maria gently guides her mother to the couch, offers a warm blanket and sits next to her, holding her hand. The physical contact and Maria's calmness seem to reassure Elena. The sundowning hasn't magically stopped and Maria still finds it very challenging, but by managing her own stress response through mindfulness and breathing techniques she is now coping with the situation much better than she did in the past.

Unlike Sally, she did not change the issue, nor did she change her perception of the issue like Jean. Instead, Maria coped with her mother's late-afternoon agitation and confusion by managing her own stress symptoms.

STAYING CALM

Máire-Anne
'There were times I found I could deal with challenging behaviour, or behaviour that was not usual from my dad, by kind of pretending that the person I was caring for was not MY dad, which funnily enough gave me a different type of patience because I had no expectation of this "person" (who was not my dad) and found I could deal with Dad's changes of behaviour in a much calmer way.'

Practical tips for coping

By consciously choosing to adopt healthier coping strategies, you can improve your ability to handle life's stresses more effectively and maintain better overall mental health. If you find yourself using coping strategies that aren't working well for you, such as avoiding issues or bottling up your feelings, try shifting to healthier methods. Here are a few practical tips to make that switch:

- **Acknowledge your feelings:** Instead of pushing your emotions away, take a moment to acknowledge them. Understanding what you're feeling can be the first step in deciding how to effectively address those emotions.
- **Seek solutions:** If you're avoiding problems, start small by tackling one issue at a time. Breaking problems down into manageable parts can make them less overwhelming and easier to handle.
- **Ask for help:** Sometimes, sharing your concerns with a friend, family member or a professional can offer new perspectives and solutions you hadn't considered.
- **Practise relaxation techniques:** Deep breathing, mindfulness and meditation are techiques that can reduce stress and improve your ability to cope with challenges.
- **Stay active:** Physical activity is a great way to reduce stress. Even a short walk can lift your mood and clear your mind, helping you to approach problems with a fresher perspective.

When care partners use problem-focused coping, their mental health will benefit and their relative will have notably slower progression of their dementia symptoms, including slower declines in their cognitive function (for example, memory) and everyday function (such as dressing, washing, eating).

Care partners can use a problem-focused approach to identify solutions to specific challenges, test these solutions and adapt their strategies based on the outcomes, thereby effectively managing their caregiving responsibilities and improving both their own and their loved one's quality of life. Problem-focused coping is associated with the best outcomes for care partners. With a specific problem in mind, the best thing is to try to seek a solution. Begin by looking at it from an objective perspective. List possible solutions – add suggestions from this book to your list as well any potential solutions suggested by others. Here are some examples of potential solutions to commonly encountered problems.

Difficulty remembering to take medications

Try technology:

- Smartphone or tablet reminders with alarms that notify both you and your relative.
- Medication apps that track doses and times, with notifications for missed doses.

Medication organisers:

- A pill organiser with compartments for each day and time (morning, afternoon, evening). Your local pharmacist may even prepare these for you.
- An automated pill dispenser that dispenses the correct dose at the right time with a sound or light alert.

Visual cues:

- Place a written or color-coded schedule for medications in a visible location, like on the fridge or next to the dining table.

Routine:

- Set a routine where medications are tied to specific daily activities (e.g. taking pills after breakfast or brushing teeth).

Professional help:

- Consult with a pharmacist or healthcare provider about simplifying the medication regimen, such as combining doses or changing to once-daily medications.

Resistance to bathing

Make sure your relative is comfortable:

- Is the bathroom warm enough? A cold bathroom might be distressing or uncomfortable.
- Try a shower chair or handheld showerhead to make the process less physically stressful.
- Offer a robe or blanket before and after bathing.

Make it enjoyable:

- Play their favorite music or calming music.
- Chat about other things during the process to distract from any anxiety they may have over bathing.
- Try scented soaps, shower gels or bath products that they find pleasant.

Routine:

- Shower or bathe at the same time every day or week, creating a predictable schedule.
- Ask yourself whether your relative needs to bathe or shower every day.
- Avoid bathing when the person is tired or agitated, as this may increase resistance.

Respect privacy and modesty:

- Allow them to bathe themselves as much as possible to maintain dignity.
- Use a large towel or bathing cape to cover areas of the body while assisting.

Offer choices:

- Give them options. Let them choose the time of day, the products they want to use, or whether they prefer a bath or shower.

Gentle encouragement:

- Use positive language, like 'Let's freshen up for the day,' instead of framing it as a chore.

Professional assistance:

- Consider involving a trained caregiver or nurse for bathing if resistance is strong, physical and/or persistent.

Try one solution from the list. Take time to objectively evaluate it. How well did it work? Did it work at all? Did it make the problem worse? If the solution is not effective, then test out another potential solution from your list. Keep trying until you find one that works or reduces the impact of the problem.

Counting your blessings is a useful way to cope that helps switch your focus to things you can be grateful for, even if it's simply something like hearing birdsong or being able to walk or feeling the sun on your face.

Perhaps a combination of solutions is what is needed. If nothing seems to make a difference, then you may have to accept that the problem cannot be solved; but taking action to find a solution may help to change your attitude to the problem and give you confidence to tackle other challenges. Many people accept defeat without even trying to find a solution. Keep experimenting and keep looking out for solutions. Caring for someone with dementia is not easy, it's challenging and at times utterly overwhelming. Every situation is unique and different strategies will work for different people.

Specific issues that you might encounter regularly, such as dealing with challenging behaviours and coping with memory loss, are covered in section 3.

CHAPTER 6

Reward

ARTHUR AND MARY

'At first it was really hard – I think we were both in shock. But once we got our heads around the disease, we just kind of got on with it. Well, after some tears we did. But there's no use crying over spilled milk, is there? We've always been active doers when faced with life's challenges so we agreed that this shouldn't be any different.

'At the beginning we treated Mary's dementia like a new project. We read everything we could about the disease and how it progresses. We didn't skim over the tough stuff; instead, we created a solutions file to have at the ready to help us to cope with a whole range of things that might arise over the course of our dementia journey. Most of these never came to pass, but knowing that we were prepared and had options that we had worked on together helped immensely. To be honest, Mary's dementia gave me a sense of purpose.

'After an initial blip immediately following diagnosis, when we were both immobilised by shock and possibly depression, we got back into our everyday rhythm. I say blip, but at the time it felt more than that and it did take us some time to regain our rhythm. We had our date night every week and hosted Sunday lunch for the family. Our adult children really rallied: they helped with housework and took Mary out a lot so that I had plenty of time for myself. They even made sure that I got to football matches with my pals. We were always a close family, but Mary's dementia brought us even closer and made us treasure our time together. I remember lots of laughing and there were tears too, sometimes both together.

> 'Mary still met her friend Camilla for coffee on Thursdays. Of course, as the disease progressed, we adjusted little things. I'd walk with Mary to the bus and wait until it arrived, make sure she had her bus pass ready, giving a nod to the driver to keep an eye out for her. Camilla would be waiting at the bus stop in town and after coffee would make sure Mary got on the right bus home and I'd meet her at the bus stop, and we'd walk back to the house together. With time we moved from using public transport to giving Mary lifts into town and eventually Camilla would come to the house for coffee instead.
>
> 'We decided early on that we wouldn't lie down to the disease but would instead do everything we could to get the most out of life and that's what we did, and it worked for us. In a way I felt a new lease of life. I felt physically strong and I had a focus that I hadn't felt since before I'd retired. I was very determined to make the best of a dreadfully difficult situation. I got great satisfaction out of figuring things out as we went along. In fact, I was quite surprised at how well I coped. I think being a doer helped.
>
> 'If I'd stopped too long to think about it, I would have drowned in sorrow or disintegrated. Instead, we kept busy and did a lot of smiling, hand-holding and hugging, but we'd always done that. Of course, eventually the disease did take over, but it never took Mary away from me. We'd been married sixty years, so we'd long ago learned to speak to each other without words. Right till the end I felt the warmth of her love.'

Purpose, reward and meaning

Arthur and Mary's story is exceptional. If, like many carers, you muddle along, more often than not just managing to keep your head above water, it's hard to imagine everything going swimmingly. But hard as it might be to believe, some care partners, like Arthur, experience growth and find that their life is enriched by dementia caregiving. People who find caregiving rewarding and enjoy positive consequences generally feel a sense of personal achievement and gratification from caregiving. They also experience feelings of mutual benefit between themselves and their relative. They speak of personal growth and finding purpose in life. In addition, they enjoy that their family is functioning well and is more united because of caregiving. My family completely fell apart but that was probably more to do with being dysfunctional in the first instance, with dementia being the catalyst rather than the cause of our family's dissolution. Many feel healthier, I didn't. They are also less bothered by the behavioural symptoms of dementia than care partners with a less positive view of their situation. Personally, I found the behavioural symptoms easy to cope with and I do think that is because I understood them, which is why I go to such lengths in this book to help you to understand them too. In addition, the people in the care of those who find dementia rewarding are less likely to be institutionalised. I share Arthur and Mary's story in the hope you can take something away that moves the 'impact of caring' dial from overwhelm and distress closer to growth and well-being.

While stress explains many of the negative health consequences of caregiving, it doesn't really explain why some care partners experience positive health effects. It could be that the physical and mental demands of caregiving help to maintain health, or that feeling appreciated by the care recipient and having a sense of purpose in life impart health benefits, or possibly it could be that adults who are healthy to begin with are more likely to become care partners. In all probability, the health rewards of positive caregiving are a combination of all three.

Arthur and Mary were very fortunate in that they had the social support of their family and friends. It's easier to be positive about a difficult situation with social support. Practical support, such as help with housework and other tasks, reduces burden, but emotional support seems to be key to having a positive view of caregiving. Having emotional support reassures, encourages and inspires care partners as they adjust to the demands of caregiving and become more accomplished care partners while they accumulate more successful experiences.

Optimism

The difficulty in dementia caregiving comes not only from the actual stressors that care partners face but also from how care partners interpret the situation. How you perceive caregiving is an important factor in determining the degree to which you experience caregiving as burdensome or beneficial. How you think about the future and your belief in your ability to take action to shape that future are both important.

Some dementia symptoms – such as sexual disinhibition, swearing, agitation, aggression and delusions about infidelity or persecution – present the greatest difficulty, making it more likely that you, the care partner, will experience burden, disstress and depression. How you view these symptoms really matters. Optimism acts as a buffer between how you perceive challenging behaviours and depression, reducing the negative consequences of caregiving and giving your well-being a boost to boot.

Optimism and pessimism are ways of thinking about the future that run along a range of positive or negative outcomes. We all have rose-tinted, blue-sky days where we feel highly optimistic about everything and everyone, and what I call low-ceiling days where clouds descend and we can see nothing but doom and gloom. But optimism and pessimism refer to your general world-view – your tendency to describe the glass as half full or half empty.

In general terms, optimism is associated with better health and a longer life. Your attitude influences how resilient you will be, especially when bad things happen. Optimists tend to be tougher, more persistent and stronger in the face of adversity.

Optimists tend to bounce back from bad experiences because they see a single setback rather than a final defeat. Optimists also tend not to generalise from the specific to the universal. By that, I mean they tend to see a 'one-off' barrier where a pessimist will see something that will undermine everything they try to do going forward. Optimists are less likely to blame themselves than pessimists. This means that pessimists often quit, stop trying and lose hope, which can lead to depression.

Control

Optimists tend to see the centre or source of control within themselves while pessimists tend to see control as lying with others or with factors external to them. People who believe that control lies within feel in control of their own destiny and see themselves as playing a very active role in their successes and failures and in shaping their life events. They believe in their own ability to shape their future and influence their environment and the people around them.

In contrast, people who see the source of control outside themselves tend to see events as passively happening to them, determined by luck, fate or chance. People who see control as something external tend to be prone to anxiety, while people who feel control within tend to be happier, less stressed and less depressed. If you lack a natural tendency towards optimism, don't worry – it can be learned. It just requires some conscious mindful effort.

What you can do

If you tend towards a glass-half-empty attitude, you might try prioritising working on cultivating a more optimistic outlook to your caregiving role. If your default tendency is to place power and control in others' hands in a resigned 'what can I do?' sort of way, you may well benefit from actively working to acknowledge that there are many more things that are within your control than you tend to think. Of course, many of life's stressors are indeed beyond your control, but adjusting how you think about them and focusing on the things you can control can help you to cope in ways that are less detrimental to your health.

Practical tips to find caregiving rewarding

The tips that follow include some practical actions that will help you to shift from an external to an internal centre of control. There are also some tips to help you to become more empowered and more optimistic, to make caregiving feel less burdensome and more rewarding.

Acquire knowledge

Enhancing your knowledge of dementia and improving your caregiving capabilities will help to improve your caregiving experience. The information in this book will hopefully equip you to become a more competent and confident care partner. More specifically, the content in section 2 of this book will inform you about dementia and what you might expect as the disease progresses. The more knowledge you have, the better you will be able to plan.

You will feel a sense of accomplishment and satisfaction emerge as you work through the process and come to understand the nature of dementia. Make use of any training that is available to you locally. Use community resources. The more skilled and knowledgeable you become, the better the caregiving experience will be for both of you. Set goals for yourself. Don't be afraid to try things. You will find what works best for you through systematic trial and error.

Armed with new knowledge, you can hopefully figure out effective ways to enhance the well-being of your relative. As your competence grows, so too will a sense of achievement from managing the condition and improving your relative's well-being. The satisfaction you will get from employing your new skills and seeing your relative respond positively will give you a great sense of fulfilment.

Arthur benefited from his feelings of accomplishment and the sense of success and value that he got from coping effectively. Care partners who have higher levels of belief in their own ability to successfully manage a situation experience more gain, even if challenging symptoms increase. In addition, the more prepared a care partner feels, the more positive their caregiving experience.

Even though you may find caregiving challenging, try to view the experience as an opportunity to explore your own ability to overcome life's challenges. But make sure you set limits that allow you to balance your caregiving demands with your own life – just as Arthur made time for football.

Shift your perspective

Dementia care partners who view dementia caregiving as an uplifting experience begin by accepting the dementia diagnosis and their associated caregiving situation. You may feel that you have no choice, and that you are stuck in a situation that was thrust upon you, but the fact of the matter is that you always have choices. You can choose to seek help and you can choose to change how you think about your situation, even if you cannot change the situation itself.

What we think determines how we feel. It is a commonly held misconception that our emotional responses are a direct consequence of an event. However, it is how you think about the event, how you appraise the event, that determines how you feel. Events don't make us sad, angry, happy or guilty – it is our interpretation of the event that influences our emotional response. An event can be anything: your relative asking you the same question for the 20th time, a sibling criticising your caregiving, your relative calling you by another name. You may not be able to change what happens, but you have the power to choose how you react to the event. Monitoring your thoughts and distinguishing helpful from unhelpful thoughts is a first step in changing how you think. The good news is that changing unhelpful thoughts into helpful ones will make you feel better. Negative thoughts can make us feel bad. By changing your thoughts, you may change how you feel. You can choose to shift from framing the situation as problematic to simply seeing it as something that just is, something that you accept. Try some of the cognitive restructuring techniques in Chapter 1.

Examples of unhelpful thinking include:

- If I don't do it, no one else will.
- No one can care for Dad as well as I do.
- Mum seems so unhappy; I must be doing something wrong.
- Maybe the doctors made a mistake and my husband will get better.
- My relative's diagnosis has destroyed my life.
- I need to put their care above my own needs.
- I need to be there for them 24/7.
- No one understands how hard being a care partner is.
- I have no time for myself, no time to socialise.

Examples of helpful thinking include:

- When my own needs are met, I can provide better care.
- Dementia is not anyone's fault.
- I can still have a meaningful relationship with my relative.
- It's OK to take time out to socialise and look after my appearance.
- Asking for help is sensible.
- Sharing my feelings will help me to manage stress.
- I don't have to let others have their way all the time.

Your attitude can have a huge influence on your stress levels. One crucial tip is to become conscious of the language you use. We all have a voice inside our head. We all engage in self-talk. Is your inner voice generally negative? Do you constantly tell yourself that you can't cope? Make an effort to notice when you are self-critical, try to stop using negative language and try to make your self-talk more positive. Instead of saying 'I can't cope', try saying 'This is really challenging but I choose not to become stressed by it. I will seek solutions, I will ask for help, I will find ways to cope.'

How you view the stressful situation rather than the situation itself determines whether it becomes an insurmountable mountain or a manageable molehill. With a little practice you can train yourself to get into the habit of substituting negative and defeatist self-talk with positive affirmative thoughts to reframe the stressor as non-threatening.

Become aware of your stressors. The Stress Log that you completed on page 76 will help you to acknowledge your stressors and your emotional response to them. Distinguish between situations and stressors you can control and those you cannot. As you work through this book, you will come to understand that you can control more than you think.

Nonetheless, there are some stressors that you must accept as being beyond your control. Reframing stressors associated with dementia caregiving requires that you shift your perspective to view challenges in a more positive or empowering way. This will help you to cope with stress and improve your overall caregiving experience. For example, handling repetitive questions from your relative can be both frustrating and exhausting. Reframing this repetition as an opportunity for you to reassure and connect with your relative can make a world of difference.

Instead of viewing the repetitive interaction as a source of frustration, you could view it as a moment of engagement. Try to see it as a way for you to provide stability and love in what is a changing and often confusing world for them. Reframing a situation doesn't belittle the reality of the stress but it can help you, the care partner, to focus on the positive impacts you are making in your relative's life.

Negative thinking can be both a source and a consequence of stress and is a common symptom of anxiety. Practising positive thinking helps to reduce stress. Try writing out your negative thoughts. The simple act of putting them on paper may free up your brain, leaving room for more positive appraisals. Avoid being self-critical and try to focus on your successes and things that you are good at. It's always important to forgive yourself when you make mistakes, lose patience or feel angry. Try to avoid pinning negative labels on your own emotions and behaviours or on aspects of your caregiving situation.

Focus on what is possible *now*. Try not to ruminate about what once was. Instead, remind yourself of the person with dementia's preserved abilities and focus on what is now possible and not on what has been lost. Remember, your relative is not their disease. They still experience fears, hopes, desires and emotions. They still want to laugh and enjoy life. Don't be afraid to laugh with them and create opportunities for fun.

Cultivate optimism

Some people have optimism-pessimism 'set points' where they consistently lean towards one extreme or the other. A healthy dose of optimism tempered with some plain old realism has genuine health benefits. While it is beneficial to cultivate optimism, it shouldn't be confused with a need to completely erase pessimism.

There is a fine balance between optimism and pessimism that holds the key to successfully navigating the world in a way that allows you to face challenges without being reckless or learn from adversity rather than being defeated and immobilised by it.

Your point of view can be trained. The way to do this is to notice when you think about caregiving as negative and instead try to focus on the positive aspects. Become aware of the voice in your head and monitor your thinking. What stories are you using to 'explain' the events unfolding in your life? The stories we tell ourselves are hugely influential. The great thing about them is that you are the author of your own stories. You can change them whenever you choose.

Ask yourself if you are being pessimistic. Are you catastrophising in your inner story? Are you blaming yourself to the exclusion of all other causes? Check your thoughts and try to consciously reframe them in a more positive light. This doesn't mean that you have to ignore difficult or unpleasant things. Rather, it means making a choice to find solutions or change your perspective or your internal dialogue despite the challenges that dementia caregiving brings.

Humans have a natural, inbuilt tendency to notice the negatives in life because they may represent danger. While this adaptive behaviour can save our life when we are actually in danger, it can lead us down a path where we fail to notice any positives in life. You can train a more optimistic outlook by making a point of noticing and holding on to positives throughout your day. It can be something really simple, like noticing the blue sky above in the morning and pausing for a moment to look at it. Or noticing a flicker of a smile on your relative's face in response to something you said or did.

Make a point of noticing positives using all your senses – hearing, sight, smell, taste, touch – five to ten times a day. Notice the world around you. Hear the rhythm of the rain tapping against the window, admire the vibrant colours on an autumn day, smell the rich aroma of freshly brewed coffee in the morning or feel the comforting warmth of a sunlit room. Relish the taste of a well-cooked meal. Pause to pet a dog or listen to a child's laughter or savour a sunset. The possibilities are endless if you take the time to notice. Engaging your senses in this way can significantly uplift your mood and positively enhance your perspective. Of course, none of these things will change the challenges you face with dementia caregiving, but it will help to train your brain to see and experience the world in a more balanced way.

Take control

You can shift your attitude and sense of control by watching your language and recognising that you can exercise choice. When you hear yourself say

'I have no choice', question it. Have you explored the options? Do you really have no other option? It can help to ask others for ideas. Sometimes we can control more than we realise, even in a situation where there really is only one option available. Even in scenarios where our choices seem limited, we often have more influence and control than we might initially think.

> ### PETRA AND IVANA
>
> Petra has spent several years caring for her mother, Ivana, who has advanced dementia. The care required is intensive and, given her mother's condition, the options available to Petra are reduced. Petra's mother can't be left alone due to safety concerns, and professional care facilities are beyond their financial means. Petra could take on the role of full-time carer or leave her mother without the support she desperately needs. For Petra, that was the same as having no choice.
>
> Initially, Petra could see only the restrictions this situation imposed on her life. Her career had to be put on hold, her social life has dwindled and her personal time is almost non-existent. She understandably felt that she had no choice in the matter, which might have led to feelings of resentment and helplessness.
>
> However, Petra decided to reframe her situation. Instead of thinking 'I have no choice', she adopted the mindset: 'I choose to care for my mother because she once cared for me, and this is my time to give back. I will use this experience to grow closer to her, to learn patience and compassion, and to develop skills I never knew I had.' By doing this, Petra has found a sense of agency in her decision. She sought out a support group for carers, where she has made new friends and learnt strategies for coping. She also documents her journey, finding moments of joy and humour amid the challenges, which she shares with others in similar situations through a blog.
>
> In reframing her limited choices as a deliberate decision to do what is best for her mother and herself, Petra has discovered a way to accept and find value in her demanding role. Her choice has become a source of strength and personal development.

While lots of things in life and in dementia caregiving are beyond your control, adjusting your attitude can help you to cope with them, freeing you up to focus on the things you can control. A realistic view of what you can and can't control, coupled with a belief that control comes from within, can make you feel empowered and emboldened to set goals and take on challenges, both of which enhance the quality of your life and caregiving experience.

Find meaning

Actively looking for benefits in your caregiving is one way to find meaning. Take some time to consider your current narrative around caregiving. What story do you tell yourself or others around what brought you to your caregiving role? Is your story simply a list of events? What story do you tell of your current experience? Does your story focus on your relative? Do you play a central role? Are you the hero or the victim in your story? Are you powerful or helpless, happy or sad? Do you create a divide between life before and after dementia? 'My life was good and now it's bad,' for example.

Perhaps you say life was great before your wife got dementia, you were really enjoying retirement, something you'd looked forward to after a lifetime of hard work. Now it's 'terrible' because of the dementia. Remember, this is *your* story. You are the author. You can tell it whatever way you want, even within the constraints of the fact of dementia. Could you, for example, retell your story by saying that retirement wasn't all it was cracked up to be? There is only so much sport you can watch on TV. It had all become a bit meaningless. I missed the challenge of work and, if I'm honest, life in general was starting to feel a bit pointless. I'd lost a sense of purpose. The dementia has changed that and I now feel I have a purpose in life. My wife really needs me and thankfully I have the resources to be a really good care partner and help her to live the best life she can with dementia. My life is challenging but I have purpose and my life has a new meaning.

Nurture your relationships

If dementia symptoms are making it hard for you to maintain a mutual, intimate, engaging relationship with your partner or parent, it is really important to pay particular attention to subtle positive responses and interpret them as conveying love, appreciation and affection. This approach will serve as a means to enhance the quality of your changing relationship.

Your relationship may change dramatically, but simply being grateful for your relative's presence and appreciating the enduring intimacy of your relationship may help. Focusing on the belief that the person with dementia would do the same for you can help too. Try to see your caregiving role as an opportunity to return the love and affection you received from the person with dementia across your life. Consider your role as a means to help maintain their identity and a way to develop a closer relationship with them. Doing all of this may also have the positive benefit of protecting you from future guilt.

Try to look beyond the caregiving difficulty and see the experience as an opportunity to enhance your relationship with your wider family as you work together to care for your relative. Embrace the mutual support that you can share with family members as you cope with the experience together. I am acutely aware that this is not possible for everyone but if you don't have the support of family, try not to dwell on it. If family becomes a source of stress, make sure you take action to protect yourself, even if that means distancing yourself from them.

It is really important to maintain your relationship and closeness with your relative despite the disease. This will likely be easier if your relationship was good prior to diagnosis. But I can tell you from my own experience with Mum that relationships can change for the better too. Dementia can be a great spur to dispense with baggage and just enjoy the moment.

There are so many ways that we can communicate love and enjoy a mutually beneficial relationship, even in the absence of language or shared memories. Dementia brings you face to face with the fragile and unpredictable nature of life. Taking some time out to take stock of your priorities may help you to place more value on the relationships that remain.

Section 1: Summary

Key messages

- Self-care is not self-indulgent – it's good self-judgement.
- Dementia caregiving has been associated with psychological benefits and better physical health for the care partner.
- Dementia caregiving can also lead to a number of negative health outcomes and can take its toll on family life and relationships.
- The burden that a care partner experiences is not directly related to the amount of work they have to do as a carer.
- The negative health outcomes associated with caregiving are most probably a consequence of chronic stress.
- Dementia care partners experience more stress and poorer physical health than other care partners.
- Challenging behaviours, known as neuropsychiatric symptoms, are the factor most likely to give rise to 'caregiver burden'.
- Perceived social support is more strongly associated with health than actual support received.
- Adaptive coping strategies and sufficient social support can lead to more positive health outcomes for the care partner.
- Constructive coping strategies are also associated with slower dementia progression in the care recipient.
- Giving and receiving support are both associated with health benefits and alleviate the negative effects of stress.
- Care partners who accept the dementia caregiving situation and adjust their perception of it to a more uplifting perspective have a more positive caregiving experience.
- Care partners who experience caregiving as rewarding set limits that allow them to balance their caregiving demands with their own life.
- Optimism in the care partner boosts well-being and reduces the negative consequences of caregiving.

Practical tips

- Set boundaries to create balance between caregiving and the rest of your life.
- Protect some personal time for yourself every day.
- Take time off without feeling guilty.
- Delegate.
- Join a care partners' support network.
- Make sleep a priority.
- Get out in daylight every day.
- Eat a well-balanced diet and maintain a healthy weight.
- Make time to exercise every day and sit less.
- Have fun exercising.
- Prioritise your health.
- Live in the moment.
- Use healthy behaviours to manage stress.
- Laugh.
- Be realistic about what you can achieve.
- Stay connected and resist the temptation to withdraw when stressed.
- Support others.
- Choose wisely who you spend your time with.
- Never underestimate the importance of human contact and a hug.
- Cultivate a confidant/e.
- Access supports and services.
- Acquire knowledge.
- Change your perspective.
- Cultivate optimism.
- Shift your centre of control to within.
- Find meaning.
- Nurture relationships.

SECTION 2
Still Me

I am not my dementia

'How's your dad?' I ask my old school friend. She responds, 'He has dementia.' The full stop after 'dementia' is ominous. The silence that follows those three words is filled with a facial expression that sadly says: Dad is gone, all that's left is dementia.

It breaks my heart to see people blinded by the disease to the extent that they fail to see the living, breathing, loving person who remains alive with feelings, needs, dreams and desires. It is easy to be fooled by dementia into thinking that your relative is no longer there. That their body is an empty shell. But that couldn't be further from the truth. Your relative is still very much alive, albeit disguised by disease, as Susan recalls.

SUSAN

'One day I had been trying to get my mother to go somewhere or do something, I can't even remember what – but I can remember what she said to me: 'I'm the mother, you're my child, I tell you what to do.' She was annoyed with me and maybe in her head it was 15-year-old me rather than the 50-year-old she was speaking to, but those words stick with me and made an impression on me. They reminded me that she was the person I had looked up to, who had taught me and cared for me. I could still ask her for advice, and she would still enquire after my well-being. I was to bear this in mind in many difficult situations, when I found myself lapsing into giving out, impatient mode.'

This section aims to help you to find and support that person, communicate with them and understand their dementia so that you can continue a meaningful relationship with them.

Chapter 7 focuses on some key issues that dramatically affect quality of life for the person with dementia. This chapter will help you to make more informed choices that take account of what people with dementia want and motivate you to implement small changes that will make a big difference for both of you.

Chapter 8 shares detailed information about Alzheimer's disease and other dementias: symptoms, stages, brain changes and alterations to memory and other cognitive functions. There is no reason for you to read about all of the different types of dementia; you can skip most of them and focus only on your relative's specific type of dementia. This information will give you the grounding you need to understand and implement the practical interventions described in section 3. The aim is for you to really understand your relative's dementia so that you can put it aside and instead focus fully on the person.

CHAPTER 7

See me

'I'm still me. I'm still your mum. I need your support to do things that I once did with ease, but I am not a child.' – Priya

I am not a child

It is vital to honour the person with dementia's adulthood and your relationship to them. While the disease may affect the nature of your relationship, it doesn't change the fact of that relationship. They remain your parent, partner, sibling or friend and as the disease progresses you may need to actively remind yourself of that. It is important that you interact with them and address them as you did before.

While people with dementia can present with childlike symptoms such as failure to follow instructions, repetition of questions and stories, difficulty carrying out basic tasks and difficulty expressing and understanding language, they have not reverted to being children. Neither their brain nor their sense of self has returned to that of a child. The changes that have occurred in their brain make it difficult for them to remember conversations and instructions and to access words to communicate or procedures to carry out everyday functions like dressing or turning on the TV. While their mood swings, irrationality and tantrums might remind you of a troublesome toddler, it is important to remember that deterioration of brain cells leads to malfunctions that underlie these behaviours and irrational thinking, making it hard for the person affected to make sense of the world. It's not difficult to see how all of these changes might lead to frustration and mood changes.

While a child's brain is developing, the brain of an adult living with dementia is degenerating. A developing brain can acquire new knowledge, learn from experience and make progress through trial and error. While each person is different, generally speaking as dementia progresses your relative will struggle to take in new information, build new brain connections and acquire new knowledge. Over time, repeatedly showing a child how to do something and commenting on mistakes will help to shape their future behaviour as they learn through trial and error. Sadly, due to the brain's diminished capacity to learn, the same approach won't necessarily work for someone in the later stages of dementia.

One thing that dementia does not steal is the person's sense of being an adult. The way they are treated matters as much to them now as it did before dementia. Possibly even more now that they are vulnerable and less able to advocate for themselves. They may not be able to articulate what they are experiencing but they will be aware that you are treating them like a child and will associate you with the unpleasant feelings that generates.

The temptation to treat your relative like a child is understandable, especially if you have raised children yourself. It even feels like a loving, caring, protective thing to do. However, in doing so you might actually be making matters worse. Indeed, you may be inadvertently contributing to low mood in your relative and escalating the incidence of the very behaviours that you are finding it difficult to manage.

It is all too easy to slip into a parental tone and use childish words. Your relative will be aware when you are acting towards them in a condescending manner. Always speak to your relative as an equal and use grown-up words like underwear (not nappy, diaper or incontinence wear), bathroom (not potty), mug (not beaker) and napkin or apron (not bib). Use whatever words you would have used before dementia. It's important too to let others involved in their care know what words your relative used for everyday things. When Mum was in residential care, she struggled when people used unfamiliar phrases. The staff would often ask her if she'd like a cuppa, and having no idea what they meant, she declined. Only minutes later to say she was parched and would love a cup of tea. You see, my mum never used the term 'cuppa', so it meant nothing to her. Unfamiliar language combined with hearing loss for a person with dementia can lead to confusion and a default refusal mode, no matter what is on offer. Have an open conversation with family members, home help and any professionals involved in your relative's care to ensure they also speak to and treat your relative as an adult, using language familiar to them.

Please be patient

> 'A little bit of your patience can make the world of difference to me.' – Ibrahim

It's not easy to be patient in ordinary circumstances and can be particularly challenging when faced with some dementia symptoms. I'm not the most patient person in the world at the best of times! Sometimes, my impatience has worked to my advantage in that it spurs me on to seek solutions so that I can get a job done as quickly as my impatient self needs. However, in the context of the difficulties associated with dementia, becoming irritated, angry or – worse still – losing your temper is not helpful. In fact, it will most probably make the situation worse and increase your feelings of guilt, stress and burden.

Your relative needs you to be patient with them. While they may not be able to tell you, they will sense your impatience, your irritation and your anger, which in turn may make them feel unsafe and agitated. Consider cultivating patience as a way to take care of yourself, a way to manage your stress levels. The good news is that patience is a skill rather than an inherent trait. So, you can develop it.

First of all, you need to recognise your triggers. A common trigger for care partners is listening to your relative repeat the same question over and over. We tend to think that external events or behaviours are the cause of our impatience, but actually it is our response to those events – our thinking – that is the cause.

Using the table template on page 130, make a note of your triggers. As a first step towards cultivating patience, take some time to notice your thoughts and how your impatience rises as your relative fails to conform to your expectations. Does your impatience rise because you haven't adjusted your expectations to account for your relative's dementia? Your natural tendency will be to expect your relative to behave as they have always done, but the fact of the matter is that your expectations are no longer realistic. You need to adjust your expectations to match the new reality.

> **SUSAN**
>
> 'I would try to explain things to my mum using the same interactions as we always did as mother and daughter. We respected each other's advice and knowledge. I had to remind myself often of my mum's dementia and that trying to explain things was fruitless. My dogs reminded me of this – when they interacted with Mum, they just wanted fun and acted as they always did with her, showing her love and affection and not making any more demands of her than to throw a ball.'

Get to know your impatience. Make a note in your table of how your impatience feels for you. Do you feel agitated, tense etc.? Whichever way it manifests, no doubt you will agree that impatience feels unpleasant. The next step is to use those unpleasant feelings as a motivation to help change the way you respond to your triggers.

I'm not pretending that cultivating patience is easy. It's not, but if you take it one step at a time you can develop the skill and it can be transformative for both you and your relative.

First of all, you can take a solution-focused approach and examine whether there is anything you can do to change the trigger. If the answer is yes, then take action to do that. In section 3 you will find practical solutions for some common triggers associated with caregiving, such as dealing with repetition.

If the answer is no, then accept the trigger as part of your caregiving role and see whether you can find any good in the situation. When we are triggered to impatience, we tend to focus on the trigger to the exclusion of everything else. We only hear the repeated question or notice the endless folding or fidgeting. But the reality is that there are lots of things going on in your environment, many of which you have control over.

Finding the good requires you to consciously make a point of switching your focus away from the trigger to something else, something more pleasant, like the music playing on the radio or the taste of the fruit scone you are eating or the smell of the scented candle in the room. Finding some way to make the experience enjoyable – or at least tolerable – will feel a lot better than anger, irritation and frustration. Make a note in your table of ways that you can make the situation good – pleasant things that you can switch your focus to.

Trigger	Thoughts	Current expectations	Feelings	Realistic expectations	Good
Repeating the same questions	*Here we go again. I really wish you would stop asking me. I told you already. Why don't you listen. I wish Dad wasn't like this, it's so hard to take when he used to be so sharp.*	Dad should ask the question only once and listen to my answer.	Patient at first. Starting to get prickly. I can feel my temper rising. I feel like I'll explode the next time he asks me.	Dad forgets that he has already asked me the question, or he forgets my answer. So, he will keep on asking.	Switch focus to music on the radio, cooking smells, a pleasant activity/hobby, or focus on your breath.
More interest in sex	This is so embarrassing, Mum is 87 but acting like a lovestruck teenager. She is flirting with the doctors and I've discovered she has been buying provocative lingerie.	Mum should act her age – she never, ever spoke about sex or acted this way when Dad was alive. She is 87, she shouldn't be interested in sex.	This is mortifying. It's also really weird to think of my mum in this way and it has sparked unwelcome thoughts of my mum in sexual relationships.	Mum is behaving out of character because of changes in her brain. These changes affect her inhibitions, and while this behaviour, is not something she is doing to embarrass me or deliberately act out of line.	Remembering that Mum is still the person I care about and that this behaviour stems from her condition. Focusing on her laughter when she's happy or the moments of connection we still share. If possible, redirecting her energy into an activity she enjoys, like knitting, drawing, or listening to music. Using mindfulness techniques to ground myself and focus on a pleasant scent, sound, or physical sensation.

130 | STILL ME

You will, of course, still have unwelcome thoughts about the situation and for a time your unrealistic expectations will remain, but you can work on giving them less weight and less importance. You might find it useful to inject a little humour as you acknowledge your own thoughts – 'What am I like? Expecting Dad to remember what I just said when I know his short-term memory is shot.' With time and training, your thoughts will become more realistic and compassionate towards yourself and your relative.

Do things with me, not for me

'I feel very scared. I know that I need help with lots of things. But there are lots of things that I can still do but you won't let me. I'm afraid to say anything in case I make you cross. Instead, I swallow my pride and let your nimble hands take over. I'd rather do it myself with some assistance from you but I'm afraid to ask in case it tests your patience. I worry that if I am troublesome you will put me in a home. So, I say nothing. I feel so useless and bored. I nod off on the sofa a lot, but I'm not tired, I just have nothing to do.' – Ravi

In the introduction to this book, I spoke of my preference for the term 'care partner'. When you see yourself as a dementia carer or caregiver, there is a huge temptation to do everything for your relative. However, if you want your relative to live the best life they can with dementia then it is vital that they do as many things as possible for themselves. This may mean that you will need to support them to get started on a task – guide or talk them through it or do some of the steps for them. It is much easier for us to do things for the person with dementia because it's quicker and possibly even less messy than doing it with them. While 'doing for' rather than 'doing with' might be a more efficient way to get through everyday activities, it diminishes your relative's independence, denies them the right to contribute to their own life and is a sure way to accelerate the loss of their abilities and the progression of their dementia symptoms. In addition, the person with dementia is likely to feel frustrated, bored, dependent and even demeaned.

As dementia progresses, try to avoid taking over tasks completely. Consider introducing modifications that will support your relative to do at least part of the task independently. Mum always asked me if she could help me prepare lunch, so I involved her in preparations: sandwich making, washing lettuce or setting the table. To be honest, it might take her forever to slice some cucumber for a sandwich, but it mattered a great deal to her to help. As we sat down to eat, she'd often say 'This is lovely, I helped, didn't I,' as if to reassure herself that she had made a contribution.

No matter what the task, there are always ways that a person with dementia can contribute. Like a lot of people with dementia, my mum loved to fold things. So, when I did the ironing, I'd give her the pillowcases to fold; she also liked to pair socks, so I'd save them for her to do. She got a great sense of satisfaction from helping me out. Think about how you can partner with your relative to complete tasks rather than take over completely. For example, if your relative's hands have become unsteady, rather than spoon-feeding them, why not help to hold the bowl still or gently guide their hand towards their mouth. Section 3 outlines some tools, devices, equipment and other technologies that may support your relative to keep doing the things they want to do.

If you encourage independence, your relative's confidence and ability will increase. Helping your relative to hold on to or increase their independence will actually lower your own stress levels. Supporting them to engage in physical activity and maintain their strength, flexibility and dexterity will also help them to continue engaging in daily tasks for longer.

Abilities can wax and wane with dementia. Some days are better than others. So just because your relative can't manage a task one day doesn't mean they will never be able to do that task again. Keep trying and encouraging – they may well be able to successfully complete the same task another day. Section 3 will deal with specific strategies you can employ to compensate for memory loss and other cognitive changes.

With nothing to do, Ravi feels bored and useless. Boredom is a common and significant issue for people living with dementia, and it affects their quality of life and their well-being. Boredom can make symptoms such as agitation and depression worse. Studies have shown that engaging people with dementia in meaningful activities can significantly reduce boredom and improve overall mood and cognitive function. Personalised activities that are tailored to the patient's abilities and interests are particularly effective. Research emphasises the importance of individualised care plans that include a range of activities to match the specific interests and capabilities of the person with dementia. This approach helps to reduce feelings of boredom and also enhance engagement with life, which is so important for everyone's well-being and mood. For example, enjoying the garden, if you have one, or spending time in green spaces such as a local park or blue space such as a river, a lake or the sea, viewing or doing art, reading or being read to, listening or dancing to music, and engaging with pets all reduce boredom.

In the advanced stage of the disease, where the person with dementia may not be able to communicate verbally or move well, it is all too easy to become preoccupied with basic care such as hygiene and nutrition and forget that your relative is still capable of becoming bored and still needs opportunities to engage with life in a meaningful way. Without stimulation and engagement, your relative will become not only bored but also frustrated, distressed and possibly depressed. You may need to get more creative in your approach to activity and find ways to adapt to your relative's changing needs and the human desire to feel connected and engaged. Even though your relative may no longer be talking, you will need to 'listen' carefully to what they are trying to communicate. Watch out for subtle changes in expression, the relaxation or contraction of muscles, a furrowed brow or a hint of a smile. Be guided by these subtle signals and respond appropriately by either quitting, continuing or adjusting the activity. When carrying out basic daily activities like washing, dressing and ensuring that your relative is eating and drinking enough, try to focus on what your relative needs and wants rather than on the process. What does that mean? Take bathing your relative, for example – try to focus on making the bath an enjoyable experience, a time to relax rather than just a way to get your relative clean. Could you play relaxing music? Light candles? (You can get scented battery-operated ones now if safety is a concern.) Talk through everything as you prepare the room. Make sure the room is warm, and once you ensure that the water is a safe temperature, let your relative test it with their hand to ensure it is to their liking. As the disease progresses or if your relative has mobility issues, it might be useful to learn how to give them a bed bath safely.

I'll never forget the screams of a very old lady who was in the same ward as my mum in an acute hospital. I am not sure whether it was a care assistant or a nurse but whichever it was, they insisted on washing that woman from head to toe despite her extreme distress. They put the poor woman through this torture on a daily basis. Did she really need to be stripped of her dignity just to follow a hospital protocol that dictates that all patients need to be thoroughly washed every day? I found it incredibly distressing to witness, but I am sure that my distress was only a fraction of that felt by the woman herself.

The important thing is to find activities that engage your relative in advanced dementia with another human being through individualised care that considers failing senses as well as offering pleasant experiences through other senses. Like a lot of older people, my mum's hearing and eyesight had declined. In the later stages, she didn't want to wear her hearing aids or her glasses – come to think of it, she didn't much like wearing her dentures either. Her senses of smell and touch were still intact, so when I visited her I would encourage her to smell whatever I brought that day, whether it was a juicy pear, some chocolate or some lavender from the garden. We held hands, we hugged and we danced, albeit just with our arms when she was too weak to get out of bed, and she never refused when I offered to apply moisturising cream to her hands and arms or to gently comb her hair. Don't underestimate the power of human touch, but always look for those subtle signals to make sure your relative is enjoying the experience.

Nothing about us without us

'I'm still here. Please don't talk about me or over me, just talk to me.' – Mervyn

It is all too easy to fall into the role of decision-maker, deciding what's best for the person you care for. You mustn't forget that your relative is still entitled to make decisions. Your role as care partner is not to decide for them but rather to support them to exercise their right to decide, whether you agree with their decision or not.

It is helpful in the early stages after diagnosis to discuss and record their wishes and preferences. If that is not possible or if decline has been sudden or rapid, then remember that language is only one way that we communicate. You and other close relatives will probably know your relative better than anyone else. You will know their preferences, their strengths and their vulnerabilities. Discuss decisions with your relative, even if they cannot respond verbally. Watch closely. They may be able to communicate their wishes to you in other ways, such as through facial expression or physical gestures. If they always made their own decisions and valued having a choice, then it's only fair to assume that they retain that desire even if they have lost the usual means to express their preference.

Involve them in as many decisions as possible. Even little things like giving them a choice of what to eat or what to wear each day can restore a sense of control to their lives. Within reason, it is important that you honour your relative's choice even if it is not what you would choose for them.

Ask for your relative's opinion and really listen to their concerns. Involve them in the conversation and don't speak about them as if they were not there. Speak to them as an adult, irrespective of how much you think they understand. Ask their permission before discussing their personal or confidential information with others.

Help to give them their voice, especially when big decisions affecting them are to be made. It has always bothered me that 'family' meetings are arranged to make important decisions about the person with dementia and the only person not invited to the meeting is the person with dementia. When I asked for my mother to be included in one such meeting, the doctor at the nursing home/hospital told me it would be too stressful for her. She was aware that a meeting was taking place and knew all her family had been called in. Her behaviour and her questions told me that not knowing and not being involved was causing her great anxiety. To this day, I still believe the momentous decision that it was in my mum's best interests to live in a care home rather than in her own home with support should not have been taken without her input. Her capacity to live independently was assessed by someone appointed by the nursing home in which she resided.

People with dementia are very vulnerable. It is natural to assume that the advice that we receive from professionals prioritises the person with dementia's best interests. While this can be the case, it is not always the case. It is important to ask questions, to ask the impact of decisions and to ask for alternatives. If you feel uncomfortable, seek a second option or the council of someone you trust or an agency that advocates for those who cannot advocate for themselves.

In my mum's case no objective assessment was made of how much support she would need to stay living in her own home. She was simply assessed to see whether she could live at home alone safely or not. When it was established that she could not live at home without risk, no intermediate solution, such as in-home professional care, was considered. It became a given that she would remain in full-time care. No cost analysis was undertaken to compare the cost of residential care to the cost of in-home professional care. It bothers me hugely that the person assigned to assess my mum's capacity and needs was appointed by the private hospital/nursing home who stood to gain financially from her care. My intention is not to point fingers but rather to question the approach. Acknowledging that she would need help to live at home, I was the only one to voice her heartfelt desire to return home. When her fate was decided by vote, not only was she not in the room but she did not have a vote. Imagine your family deciding your fate without your input.

Some time later, in an effort to take advantage of a state scheme to minimise the cost of care, there was an opportunity to move Mum to a nursing home that was covered by this scheme. I received a call from a member of Mum's team asking me if I would like to view the proposed nursing home. She told me that my siblings who viewed the nursing home had deemed it suitable, but she wanted to offer me the opportunity to view it before setting the wheels in motion. When I asked her what Mum felt about the nursing home, she was dumbfounded. She told me that Mum hadn't seen it. I asked her to arrange for me to take Mum to see the place for herself, since she would be the one living there. Mum made it very clear to the team member who accompanied us that day that she didn't like the place. She was very vocal about the low ceilings, which she said made her feel claustrophobic and depressed. She also declared the décor to be dreadfully old-fashioned (it was) and far too chintzy for her taste. She actually became a bit panicky at the thought of being made to live there and so while she still really wanted to go home, she felt that if she couldn't go home then she would prefer to stay in the hospital/nursing home she had become accustomed to. Aside from coming to me at weekends and stays in acute hospital, she spent the rest of her days there, with no support from the state. Her bank accounts were emptied and her house put up for sale to cover the costs. She died on Valentine's Day 2016, the day before the contracts for the sale of her house were to be signed.

I have served on several committees for an organisation here in Ireland called Sage Advocacy, who champion the rights of vulnerable older adults. Their guiding principle, 'Nothing about you without you' is a good one to guide you when decisions need to be taken that affect your relative.

Your relative's local authority (council) may appoint an independent mental capacity advocate (IMCA) to speak on their behalf. This will happen when a major decision needs to be made, such as whether the person should move to a care home or have serious medical treatment. An IMCA is also sometimes involved if there is conflict between family members. In the UK the National Institute for Health and Care Excellence (NICE[7]) promotes the rights and interests of people who may need

---

[7] https://www.nice.org.uk/guidance/settings/care-homes.

support with decision-making, and in Ireland it's the Decision Support Service[8].

Getting in contact with your local Alzheimer's Society for advice around the time of diagnosis will help you and your relative understand how their future might be affected, make you both aware of supports and services, and help you to plan for the future. The Alzheimer's Society have dementia advisors who can help you and your relative to understand what their rights are and enable you to make informed decisions – for example, around what supports your relative might need or be entitled to. Having an independent advisor or advocate is critical when decisions are being made about long-term care, where the wishes of the person with dementia can get lost in the conflicting opinions of various family members and health professionals. If a person with dementia expresses a desire to remain at home, an independent advocate can ensure that every effort is made to support the person with dementia to do this. The costs associated with providing professional care in the home are often far less than the costs associated with residential care. Advocates can also advise the care partner, especially when it comes to taking on formal roles like power of attorney. Contact your local GP, Alzheimer's Society, local authority, health authority or Citizens Advice to find out about independent advocates and advisors.

Elder abuse

'My daughter, Claire, has put my wedding and engagement rings somewhere safe. I don't know where they are, and I really miss wearing them. I feel sad when I look at my naked fingers. I feel like I am betraying Claire's dad by not wearing them. I keep asking Claire to give me my rings. She says she will, but she never does.' – Kay

---

[8] https://decisionsupportservice.ie/home.

We tend to think of elder abuse as something that is carried out intentionally with malice, such as physical violence, sexual assault or financial abuse. But unfortunately, abuse can occur as a consequence of the well-intentioned actions of a care partner who means well but is unaware that some of the steps they have taken to protect their relative may actually constitute elder abuse.

Claire has not stolen Kay's rings. She simply made a decision to keep them safe in her own apartment after Kay mislaid them for the third time. Claire knows how important the rings are to her mum and couldn't bear to think of how distraught she would be if she lost them. However, she failed to take account of – and continues to ignore – the distress that her mum is experiencing as a consequence of not being allowed to wear her rings. Claire is also unaware that she has no right to deny her mother access to her rings, and indeed her actions could be interpreted as elder harm because she has taken her mother's property against her will and has refused to return it despite her mother's repeated requests.

It's easily done, and I believe that most care partners would be horrified to learn that their actions could be interpreted as abusive, especially as caring for a loved one with dementia is a profound act of kindness and commitment. A commitment that requires a deep understanding of both the needs of the person with dementia and the legal responsibilities involved. It's important to recognise that elder abuse isn't always intentional; sometimes our well-meaning actions can inadvertently cross boundaries, leading to serious consequences.

Elder abuse is about more than just physical harm. It includes neglect, emotional abuse, financial exploitation and more. For instance, unintentional neglect can occur when a care partner is overwhelmed and unable to provide the necessary care. Emotional abuse might arise from repeated impatience or dismissive remarks. Financial abuse could be as simple as mishandling the person's funds without realising the legal requirements for managing their money.

Educate yourself to avoid unintentional harm and understand your responsibilities better. Seek out resources that explain the signs of abuse and how to avoid them. The websites for your national health service or national Alzheimer's association will offer comprehensive guides and toolkits. By joining a care partners' support group, either locally or online, you might gain insights and emotional support that reduce the risk of 'caregiver burnout' and potential neglect or abuse.

From a legal standpoint, elder abuse is taken very seriously, and laws are strict to ensure the protection of vulnerable seniors. Each jurisdiction may have specific statutes defining what constitutes elder abuse and detailing mandatory reporting requirements. As a care partner, familiarising yourself with these laws is crucial. They are designed not only to protect the person with dementia but also to guide and protect you – the care partner and other family members – from legal repercussions. If you are unsure about your legal obligations or the right course of action in complex situations, consulting with a social worker, an older persons' advocacy group, a solicitor familiar with elder care or an Alzheimer's association can provide clarity and direction. Organisations such as NICE in the UK and Decision Support Services in Ireland give clear guidelines that support a care partner to formalise their supporting role. These guidelines are really useful even if you do not formalise your role through power of attorney, for example.

Try to remember that maintaining respect and dignity in caregiving is paramount. Regular self-reflection on your caregiving methods and the well-being of your relative can help identify potential issues early. If you find yourself feeling overwhelmed, seeking respite care or professional help is not a sign of failure but a proactive step in ensuring the best care for your relative while maintaining your own health.

If you share the responsibility of care with others, including family and paid carers, or your relative lives in a care home or spends time in hospital or respite care, it is important to keep an eye out for signs of abuse, some of which are easier to detect than others. It can be a real challenge to determine whether the first four on the following list are symptoms of dementia or signs of abuse. Remember, older people can bruise easily, but it is important to diplomatically ask your relative and those responsible for their care at the time of the injury how the bruises came about.

- Sudden changes in their behaviour – for example, being depressed, tearful or feeling helpless.

- Being quiet and withdrawn.
- Being aggressive or angry.
- Not wanting to be left alone with particular people.
- Looking untidy, unwashed or thinner than usual.
- Being unusually light-hearted, insisting nothing is wrong.
- Missing possessions.
- Changes in finances.
- Bruises, wounds, breaks or other injuries, particularly repeated injuries.

Studies suggest that up to half of people with dementia experience some form of abuse or neglect. Sadly, the complexity of their care, combined with their impaired ability to report abuse, makes them particularly vulnerable. Abuse in care homes and hospitals is also a significant concern, with estimates suggesting that about 20 per cent of nursing home residents have experienced some form of abuse. This is due to numerous factors, including lack of staff training, inadequate staffing levels and insufficient oversight.

When discussing concerns with your relative, use simple language and be patient. Ensure the environment is calm and free from distractions. Be empathetic and reassure them of their safety, which can help in gaining their trust and willingness to open up about their experiences.

If you suspect abuse, making a formal complaint is crucial. Start by speaking to the care home manager or hospital administration. If you wish to escalate an issue, care homes should nominate an independent person in the contract of care/policies to whom you can bring a complaint.

For hospitals in Ireland, there is Your Service Your Say. This national complaints and feedback system for healthcare services enables patients, families and care partners to voice concerns, offer compliments, or provide suggestions about their experiences. Operated by the Health Service Executive (HSE), it covers all public healthcare facilities, including hospitals, clinics, and community health services. The system emphasises a patient-centred approach, aiming to resolve complaints locally and efficiently. Importantly, the process upholds confidentiality and respects individuals' rights, striving to improve the quality and safety of healthcare services across Ireland. In the United Kingdom, the National Health Service (NHS) provides a structured process for patients to offer feedback or lodge complaints about healthcare services. Patients are encouraged to first address concerns directly with the service provider, such as a hospital or GP practice. Many issues can be resolved informally by speaking with the staff involved in your relative's care. If this doesn't lead to a satisfactory outcome, you can escalate the matter to the complaints manager or the Patient Advice and Liaison Service (PALS) associated with the NHS trust. PALS offers confidential advice, support, and information on health-related matters. They can assist in resolving concerns or guide you through the NHS complaints procedure.

If local resolution is unsuccessful or if you prefer to make a formal complaint, you can do so in writing, by phone, by email, in person, or using an online complaints form. Each NHS organisation has its own complaints procedure, and if you're unsure who to contact, PALS can provide guidance. This is a free and independent service that can help you make a complaint about an NHS service. They can assist with writing letters, explaining responses, and preparing for meetings. Every local authority must make this service available. It's important to note that the NHS encourages feedback to improve services, and patients have the right to make a complaint about any aspect of NHS care, treatment, or service. The NHS Constitution outlines these rights and the commitment to address complaints efficiently and transparently.

POSITIVE CHANGE

Martina

'I would say do not be afraid to complain. If you do not complain nothing will change. You are by default saying that the situation is acceptable, but if you do complain you may get positive change.'

If the issue is not resolved, you can escalate the complaint to local health authorities or regulatory bodies – for example, the Care Quality Commission (CQC – England), the Care Inspectorate (SCI – Scotland), the

Regulation and Quality Improvement Authority (RQIA – Northern Ireland) and the Health Information and Quality Authority (HIQA – Ireland). However, while they may be prompted to carry out an inspection of a nursing home on the basis of an issue being highlighted or a complaint, they will not address a particular incident or individual complaint. The Ombudsman is also an option.

If a situation arises where you feel it is necessary to remove a relative from a care home, seek legal advice to ensure all actions comply with local laws. Gather all necessary documentation and consult with your relative's healthcare provider to discuss the safest approach for their transition, especially if your relative lacks the capacity to make decisions.

KEEP A RECORD

Susan

'If you do need to complain, keep the expletives in your head or save them for the journey home in the car afterwards. Try to stay calm when facing the healthcare provider or residential care provider you are dealing with. Keep a record of conversations and dates. I would feel angry, frustrated and worried when I could not get Mom the care she needed or I felt that she had been mistreated, ignored, and her human rights had been violated. It sounds very strong, but that's what it came down to. We, as carers, are also often ignored and not listened to.

'I kept records and got as much information as I could. Sometimes I went as far as taking photos of hospital charts so I could understand what medications Mom was receiving and comparing them with her usual medication, of which I also kept a list. That enabled me to follow up with the hospital on one occasion when I noticed their failure to administer her regular heart medications for two consecutive days after being admitted for another ailment, and another time to discover the inappropriate use of psychotropic medications.

'I often sat at my desk at work worried, angry and frustrated about what was going on with Mom's care, and to deal with that, in the moment, I would write an email laying out all my thoughts, noting

> the conversations I had had and putting down the facts I could recall. The email would only ever be sent to myself. Later, when I needed to follow up in writing on complaints or concerns I had raised verbally, I would have my email notes to guide me with the facts, but the emotional, angry rant would stay with me.
>
> 'In short, write it down in an email, a notebook, a voice note, a diary. It helps organise your thoughts, get out your frustrations, and keep organised. Always follow up any complaint in writing if you can and use any of the official channels there are to escalate a complaint if necessary. If it doesn't benefit your loved one, it might help someone else. It always made me feel better to know I could do something. Mom's health was seriously affected by the administration of psychotropic medications both in hospital and in a nursing home. I managed to put a stop to their use in her case, and I have since been able to put the experience and knowledge I gained by contributing as a carer advocate to the development and implementation of the National Clinical Guideline No. 21: Appropriate prescribing of psychotropic medication for non-cognitive symptoms in people with dementia published by the Department of Health, Ireland, December 2019[9].'

I could have done with following Susan's advice over the course of my mum's journey when the way she was treated in both acute hospital and nursing home settings appalled me. But I let the anger and the expletives loose – which gave them an excuse to ask me to leave and make it look like I was the bad guy, not they who had prescribed psychotropic medications inappropriately or failed to treat Mum with dignity and respect. For example, they had refused to take Mum to the bathroom despite my pleas and those of my son, who was with me visiting Mum in her private nursing home. For safety reasons, I wasn't allowed to take Mum to the bathroom. Cutting a very unpleasant story

---

[9] *Department of Health (2019). Appropriate prescribing of psychotropic medication for non-cognitive symptoms in people with dementia (NCEC National Clinical Guideline No. 21). Available at:* https://www.gov.ie/en/collection/c9fa9a-national-clinical-guidelines/

short, Mum became increasingly distressed as she waited to be taken to the bathroom. Eventually, she soiled herself and was perfectly aware that she had. It was beyond horrific.

Balance risk and rights

> 'I hear you telling others that I'm not safe anymore. Please don't stop me from doing things just because I might forget or fall. I'd rather die from falling than from boredom.' – Julie

Taking risks is part and parcel of everyday life – take the inherent risks of burns or cuts that come with using sharp knives, hot ovens, hot pots and boiling liquids while we prepare a meal. This is something that we choose to do on a daily basis, despite the risks, because it is an essential and fulfilling activity that gives us autonomy and the satisfaction of making meals we enjoy eating. Throughout our days whether crossing the road, taking a walk or making a cup of tea we are taking some level of risk. People with dementia should have the opportunity to balance risk and quality of life. You as their care partner can support your relative to balance risk with quality of life by recognising the importance of their personal freedom and dignity. If your relative still has the capacity to make decisions, they retain the right to choose actions that might involve risk to themselves.

Everyone, including people with dementia, has the right to take risks. This is something that can be very difficult for care partners to accept. No one wants to see a relative fall or have an accident. But no one wants to live a life so risk-averse that they don't get to have any quality of life. Risk is part and parcel of life. Life is for living and no one, not even a person with dementia, wants to live it locked away from the world, in a boring bubble, wrapped in cotton wool.

As a care partner, you need to be mindful of balancing the quality of care that you provide with the quality of life that your relative experiences. If your relative does have an accident, you may be worried that you could be blamed by family members or by authorities. Try not to let this fear overly influence your choices and behaviours. There is a big difference between wilful neglect and planned care that takes into account the wishes of the person with dementia in the context of the associated risks. The table on page 130 will help you to develop a care plan around your relative's preferences and the safety issues that concern you. If the person with dementia gives permission, then share the plan with the rest of the family and healthcare professionals. A carefully constructed care plan can help to protect you should things go awry but not if you have been wilfully negligent or abusive.

People with dementia have the right to participate in decisions, particularly those that affect their human rights. Human rights apply to everyone and that includes people with dementia. Human rights are equal and cannot be placed in hierarchical order – for example, based on disability or cognitive status. Human rights cannot be given and cannot be taken away, neither can they be relinquished or traded for other privileges. Human rights are based on principles of fairness, equality, dignity and respect. When it comes to the human rights of your relative, you have rights and responsibilities.

While it is important always to consider safety, decisions made solely to eliminate risk can end up denying the person with dementia their fundamental human rights. People with dementia often want to walk about. For this reason, most residential nursing homes have closed doors to limit free movement in order to prevent their residents from getting lost and to minimise the risk of falls or accidents. This practice is so normalised that, generally speaking, people accept it as a good thing. But is it? Is locking someone away really in the best interests of the person with dementia or is it something that makes life easier for the nursing home and hospital management and staff?

When people with dementia are kept behind closed doors for safety, it restricts their freedom to move around as they choose. Studies show that this kind of restriction can harm their quality of life and sense of independence. Research also reveals that many residents in nursing homes feel frustrated when their movement is limited. This frustration can lead them to engage in resistance behaviours and show signs of distress, behaviours often labelled as 'challenging' or 'symptoms of dementia'. Unfortunately, these behaviours can then become reasons for further confinement.

There is no doubt these behaviours *are* challenging – but are they symptoms of dementia or are they simply a response to being deprived of their liberty and the right to choose what they want to do? When my mum was in an acute hospital, they also operated a closed-door policy. My mum wanted to walk – in fact, she wanted to leave the ward – but one nurse found her behaviour so 'challenging' that she sedated Mum. This type of sedation is the equivalent of restraining her physically by, for example, tying her to her chair. She literally couldn't move and was incredibly distressed because she couldn't understand why she couldn't move. She thought she'd had a stroke and couldn't understand why no one would help her. That's the stuff of nightmares. This form of sedation when used to limit the movement of patients is often referred to as a chemical straitjacket. If you are thinking this is for her own safety, think again. Yes, safety seems like a plausible justification on the surface. When you live through the situation, the stark reality of it, and see that your relative just wants to go for a walk and is severely medicated to deny her that basic right, that will change your perception pretty quickly. Closed-door policies that restrict patient freedom prioritise the financial considerations and the needs of the staff and the facility over the needs, health and well-being of the person with dementia.

Recent years have seen a move towards open- or semi-open nursing homes that afford people with dementia a level of independence and a sense of normality completely absent from the traditional nursing home. Nursing homes that embrace the desire to walk about see it simply as person-centred care – a term often used, but by traditional nursing homes rarely true to its definition. In open-setting nursing homes, people with dementia are free to choose where they walk, including outside the nursing home. In semi-open-door settings, residents are allowed to move freely within the care setting and gardens but are not allowed to enter the outside world unaccompanied.

Most of us want to spend time walking. Think back to how important a daily walk became to us during the pandemic, when our movements were severely restricted. Just like you and I, people with dementia want to spend time walking. It's good exercise and can relieve boredom and release stress. The desire to walk can increase and you may notice that your relative seems to be in perpetual motion walking around the house or care home, sometimes during the night. This desire to walk about is often referred to as 'dementia wandering', a term increasingly considered unhelpful because it suggests the person is walking with no purpose. It can be difficult to determine why your relative is walking about and it may become a problem if your relative has memory issues or cannot find their way home. With effort, it is possible to discover the reasons or beliefs behind the walking and help them to remain safe and independent. A change in your relative's walking patterns can often indicate that they have an unmet need that they cannot articulate. The 'What you can do' section at the end of this chapter offers suggestions on how you can support your relative to remain independent while balancing risk with freedom. It's not easy, but it is important.

Try to avoid being overprotective. Just saying yes can be more beneficial than being overly cautious and restrictive in terms of what your relative does or doesn't do. Acknowledge that the power to decide does not reside with you. You are a care partner who will support them to do what they desire in the safest way possible. If you do have to restrict activities, try to adopt the least restrictive approach, as outlined in the examples below.

Meal preparation

Restrictive approach: Preparing all meals for your relative because you fear they might cut or burn themselves. Or stopping your relative from from using the kitchen entirely because of safety concerns.

Least restrictive approach: Being there and keeping an eye on them while they cook, using safer tools (e.g. a microwave instead of a stove), or buying pre-prepared ingredients such as chicken pieces, or pre-cut carrots and other veg.

Socialising with friends

Restrictive approach: Discouraging your relative from attending social events because they might become confused, embarrassed or get lost.

Least restrictive approach: Arranging for someone they trust to accompany them, ensuring they have a phone or way to contact you if they need assistance.

Choosing what to wear

Restrictive approach: Insisting on deciding what they wear because they might choose inappropriate clothing.

Least restrictive approach: Laying out weather-appropriate options for them to choose from or offering subtle suggestions while allowing them autonomy.

Participating in physical activities

Restrictive approach: Not allowing them to take part in activities like gardening or light exercise because they may fall.

Least restrictive approach: Ensuring the environment is safe (e.g. removing trip hazards, providing stable gardening tools and cushioned surfaces), and being present to assist only if asked.

Handling money

Restrictive approach: Removing their access to money or bank cards out of fear they'll overspend or get scammed.

Least restrictive approach: Accompanying them when shopping, while still allowing them to make decisions. Being prepared to return goods on their behalf if they purchase something on a whim that they don't need, or already have (sometimes in multiples).

It's all about the person, not the disease – if you focus on the person, there is always some way you can make their life a little better, a little more enjoyable and a little more hopeful. But remember, doing that doesn't have to be at the expense of *your* health and well-being. Always communicate directly with your relative. Avoid the temptation to talk over them or about them as if they weren't there. It's also important not to talk down to them or at them. Very often, people with dementia understand more than they communicate and yet you may encounter doctors and other health professionals who will talk over the patient with dementia, directing their attention to you. Remind these people that your relative is in the room and tell them that you would like them to communicate directly with your relative – with both of you. If you are not sure how much your relative understands it's best to assume they understand everything.

Being aware of legal frameworks is important when supporting a relative with dementia. Laws like the Mental Capacity Act (England and Wales), Assisted Decision-Making Act (Ireland), Adults with Incapacity Act (Scotland), and Mental Capacity Act (Northern Ireland) emphasise supporting individuals to make their own decisions wherever possible. They promote dignity, rights, and the least restrictive options while guiding care partners on how to: assess capacity, act in the person's best interests, and seek legal authority when needed. For further information, consult your local Alzheimer's Association or the relevant legal guidelines in your region.

In the initial stages, your relative may deny diagnosis and minimise symptoms. This is different from a patient's lack of awareness of their condition and symptoms, which likely occurs when the disease is much further progressed at the time of diagnosis. When patients are aware but choose to deny for a period of time, try to be wary of stripping away what may be a useful defence mechanism while they come to terms with the diagnosis.

MATTEO, ENZO AND LUCIA

Matteo noticed that his father, Enzo, recently diagnosed with early-stage Alzheimer's, consistently downplayed his forgetfulness and insisted nothing was wrong, despite clear evidence of memory lapses. Understanding his father's need to maintain a sense of control and normalcy, Matteo chose a gentle approach. He initiated conversations about ways to support daily tasks without directly confronting the Alzheimer's diagnosis. For example, he introduced a digital calendar to help his father manage appointments and tasks, which his father considered a tool for efficiency rather than a coping mechanism for his condition.

This worked well and encouraged Matteo to come up with other ways to implement small but effective supports to help Enzo manage the challenges of early-stage dementia while respecting his desire for independence and control. Matteo checked in with his dad regularly via phone calls or visits, which eased Matteo's concerns about his father's well-being but also provided companionship and emotional support for Enzo during a difficult time.

Since the death of Matteo's mum, Enzo had been coming to Matteo and his wife Lucia's house for Sunday lunch. Lucia never needed an excuse to shop so she did some searching online and found some cute but useful items that she and Matteo thought would help Enzo. She bought two sets of every item. She placed one in her home and had a spare at the ready to gift to Enzo when he noticed the item or when she told him how useful it was. She found a pictorial reminder for *keys – wallet – glasses – phone* online for her hall door, which she bought with Enzo in mind but has actually found to be a really useful reminder for herself. Lucia moved a quirky big mouth hippo ornament she'd received as a gift but never quite known what to do with into a place for wallets, glasses, keys and anything else the family seemed to misplace regularly. She encouraged Enzo to deposit his keys there when he came to visit. After a few weeks, she gifted Enzo a large frog she'd bought online with a gaping mouth similar to her hallway hippo. She suggested he use it to store his keys, wallet, glasses, etc.

These small, subtle supports not only helped Enzo to cope with daily tasks but also boosted his confidence and ability to manage his own care as much as possible. Over time, this and other small supports helped Enzo gradually acknowledge his challenges in a non-threatening way, allowing him to accept more targeted interventions as his needs changed. By maintaining a sensitive approach and supporting independence, you can help your relative adjust to the reality of their condition at their own pace, without overtly challenging their initial defence mechanisms.

What you can do

Ensuring that your relative maintains independence for as long as possible is key, but it's natural to worry about the potential for harm. When the person is inclined to walk about, it's important to strike a balance between supporting their freedom and keeping them safe.

Everyday life will always involve some level of risk, and deciding what's acceptable is a conversation that includes the person with dementia and anyone involved in their care. This shared understanding supports their quality of life while preserving their independence and dignity.

If the person still has the capacity to make decisions, they retain the right to choose actions that might involve risk to themselves. Having said that, while it is important to give your relative autonomy to choose risk, the risk to others must also be considered. For example, your relative may choose to drive but their ability to do so safely would impact the safety of others.

When capacity is no longer present, it remains essential to involve them in discussions about their care to the extent they're able. In all cases, decisions should be guided by what is genuinely in their best interests and that means considering their mental health and psychological well-being as well as their physical safety and the safety of others.

How you approach their safety will depend on your relative's ability to manage on their own and why they may be prone to walk about. Consider if their surroundings are suitably safe and whether adjustments could reduce any potential hazards. While no environment is ever entirely risk-free, some are certainly safer. For example, a familiar, quiet neighbourhood where the person is well known may present fewer risks. Examining their surroundings with this in mind can help in finding ways to minimise hazards.

If your relative feels the need to walk, try to support this safely by first understanding the reasons behind it and what they need. Walking may simply be a phase they go through but the more you understand their need to walk, the better you will be able to support them safely.

Observe their walking habits and take notes for a few weeks. What is happening in their surroundings before they go walking, what is their behaviour when they go walking? Write down whatever you notice and include any reasons they give for walking or anything they say when they go walking. Tedious as it may sound, it may help you to identify triggers or patterns.

Make sure your relative has somewhere safe to walk at home. Does the house have a garden? If so, make sure it is safe to walk in, with a clearly defined level path to follow. Remove potential trip hazards and make sure the surface is not slippery by regularly clearing moss, lichens and algae. Consider adding a handrail along the path and places of interest to stop, sit and linger. The garden doesn't have to be huge to add a bird feeder, fairy garden, sundial, outdoor ornaments or a small bench in a sunny or shady spot. Remember the importance of the sense of smell and include plants like lavender or scented roses by seating areas.

If neither you nor your relative have a garden, make it part of their daily routine to walk in the local park or nearest green space. Do some research: there may be a local service, organisation or informal group that supports people with dementia to stay active by organising group walks or other leisure and well-being activities. Joining a local dementia café might help you both connect with others in similar situations who know about groups, or perhaps you could join forces and create your own local walking group.

Some communities are very dementia aware and have schemes in place to help ensure the safety of local residents with dementia. Contact your local council to establish whether there is a Neighbourhood Return scheme in your area. These schemes involve volunteers who help local residents with dementia return home safely and also help to look for people with dementia who may have become lost.

Rather than trying to stop your relative from walking, try to support their desire to walk. Try not to argue – even rational explanations as to why you want to prevent them from walking could be very upsetting for them. The best thing to do is see if you can find out from them where it is they want to go. Help them prepare to go walking safely. For example, make sure they are wearing the right kind of clothes and shoes for walking, whatever the season. If you can go with them, then do. Once you have walked a while, you can try to distract them and guide them back home safely. This approach has better outcomes than preventing them or arguing with them. If you are not in a position to go with them, consider asking relatives or friends to accompany your relative.

From a safety perspective, it is really important that your relative carries some form of identification with them. This doesn't have to be a formal, important document like a passport, driver's licence or identity card – it could simply be a handwritten card with the name and phone number of someone who can be contacted should they get lost, or a piece of engraved jewellery or a smartwatch your relative is happy to wear. The card could be popped into the pockets of clothing, or even sewn in to clothing or a bag or stuck on the back of a phone or some other item they reliably take with them. Contact the Alzheimer's Society for free 'helpcards' on which emergency contact details, your relative's name and a note of things they need help with are written. If your relative has a mobile phone and reliably takes it with them, adding a tracking app could be useful, but this can only be used with the consent of your relative.

You could also speak to your neighbours and other members of your community such as the local shop, post office, police station, coffee shop. Discreetly tell them about your relative's needs, share your contact details and ask them to keep an eye out for your relative's safety and to call you if they are concerned. Again, you need to have your relative's permission before you disclose to other people that they have dementia. If your relative doesn't have the capacity to give consent, you need to think carefully whether telling other people is in your relative's best interests.

Everyone involved in your relative's care, including paid in-home carers, should be encouraged to support your relative's need to walk about. If you are using day care, respite care or are considering long-term nursing home care, it is important to establish their policy around walking and closed doors to inform your decision and ensure that those policies genuinely have your relative's best interests at the core.

It can be really hard to know how to find the right balance between risk, liberty, safety and independence, especially when your relative wants to leave the house. Yes, you can support them by going with them, but this might not always be possible or the desire to walk might occur very frequently. In these cases, you can try to encourage them to stay at home by offering them an activity to do. Try to focus their attention on something else. Even tasks that seem mundane to you, like folding the ironing or pairing socks, can help to divert your relative's attention, especially if boredom is at the root of their desire to walk. You may increase your likelihood of success by suggesting activities that involve movement, such as dancing or sweeping the floor.

If you are concerned that your relative may leave the house without you knowing, it might be helpful to install a door sensor that will alert you and anyone else caring for your relative when they open the front door. There are lots of smart technologies that can help – again, I must reiterate, especially when it comes to tracking or monitoring devices, that these should only be employed with your relative's consent. If your relative genuinely doesn't have the capacity to consent in a meaningful way then only proceed if you honestly know it is in your relative's best interests.

Locked doors

Locking doors may seem like an obvious and simple solution to prevent your relative from coming to harm, but a person with dementia – or indeed any person at all – should not be locked in when they are alone. A locked door, including a locked bedroom door, can leave the person with dementia trapped if there is a fire. If they have an accident or fall then locked doors can make it difficult for help to access them or for them to access help. Locking a person in may cause them to panic and go to dangerous lengths to free themselves.

Of course, locking our main house doors at night is advisable for all of us for safety and security reasons. My concern lies with locking doors in such a way that only you, for example, have the key to unlock it, leaving others without a key completely trapped. Doors can be locked and made safe from the inside with bolts etc. that can be opened. If you or someone else is in the house with your relative and the front door leads on to, say, a busy road or a dangerous balcony, then it may be acceptable and genuinely in your relative's best interests to lock the door. If your relative has the capacity to make the decision, you can lock the door with their consent. It is important to discuss these issues with everyone and anyone involved in your relative's care. If your relative lacks capacity, it may be possible to make the decision on their behalf. But remember, locking a door deprives your relative of their liberty, so it would be wise to speak to social services before any such decision is taken, even where you have your relative's best interests at heart. Social services may want to make an independent assessment of the situation.

> **SUSAN**
>
> 'Mum used to wander a lot at night. I found that locking the kitchen (I was in the habit of doing it anyway, because the cats can open the door) where all the dangerous things like cleaning products, knifes etc. were, reassuring because she only had access to the "safe rooms" at night.'

Susan's approach – locking the kitchen door at night – is a good example of how to keep your relative safe without compromising their freedom. In contrast, locking your relative's bedroom to prevent them from having an accident during the night might be well-intentioned, but the truth is that it deprives them of their liberty and turns their bedroom into a prison cell. The mental distress that causes each and every night must be weighed against the risk of falling.

Here are some alternative strategies, informed by research, for supporting the safety of your relative at night without resorting to locking their bedroom door:

- **Create a safe pathway with soft lighting:** Poor lighting increases fall risk among people with dementia. Research supports that night lights or illuminated pathways improve safety by reducing disorientation and supporting spatial awareness. Place soft, motion-activated lighting along pathways to the bathroom or other frequently accessed areas. This approach can reduce the likelihood of falls by providing clear visibility. I use night lights that simply plug into wall sockets in my own home to guide the way to the bathroom so that I don't have to turn on a bright light and risk waking myself up too much in the middle of the night.

- **Arrange the room for maximum safety:** Dementia-friendly environments with simple, hazard-free layouts have been found to decrease the incidence of falls and other injuries. Remove any trip hazards like loose rugs, ensure that furniture is placed out of the way, and add non-slip mats to the floor if needed. An occupational therapist can offer advice on this if you have access to one.
- **Ensure safe access to the bathroom:** Walking about at night-time is often motivated by the need to use the bathroom. Studies show that reducing the distance to the toilet can reduce both walking about and the risk of falls. Remove any barriers to bathroom access, such as obstacles in hallways, or consider providing a bedside commode if the bathroom is far away.
- **Provide reassurance through familiar items:** Familiar objects can help reduce agitation and 'wandering' in people with dementia, especially at night, by creating a more reassuring environment. Place familiar and comforting items, such as family photos or a favourite blanket, within easy reach to create a sense of security. Consider replacing glass in photo and picture frames with Perspex or plastic to avoid accidents involving broken glass.
- **Structured sleep environment and routine:** Studies highlight that regular routines can improve sleep quality and reduce the need for night-time walking about, which often arises from confusion or restlessness. Establish a consistent bedtime routine and create a calming environment. You can do this by reducing noise, playing low-level, calming music, using blackout curtains if needed, and keeping the room at a comfortable temperature, neither too hot nor too cold. The ideal temperature for inducing sleep is 65 degrees Fahrenheit (18 degrees Celsius).
- **Motion sensors or bed alarms:** Studies suggest that passive monitoring tools, like motion sensors or bed alarms, can alert care partners when the person is getting up without restricting their movement. If you live with your relative, these devices can help you respect their space and autonomy while also giving you peace of mind.

- **Monitoring technology or wearable devices:** Wearable technology has shown promise in providing unobtrusive monitoring, especially for people with dementia who walk about frequently. Such tools allow care partners to respond quickly without imposing physical restrictions. I can't say this often enough: you must have your relative's consent. Some advanced models can alert care partners to unusual movement patterns, such as prolonged periods out of bed at night.
- **If your relative goes missing:** Try to stay calm and contact the police if necessary. Keep a recent photo of your relative for identification, and consider filling out the Herbert Protocol form (herbertprotocol.com), which stores vital information to help the police if you report your relative missing. Keep someone at home in case they return and focus searches on places they've previously visited or enjoyed.

If they return home on their own, they may feel anxious, so try to offer reassurance rather than questioning them immediately. Once they're settled, gently ask where they went and why, as this can provide insights to prevent similar situations in the future. After the situation is resolved, take time for yourself. Talking to friends, family or a professional can be helpful in managing any stress or anxiety following the event.

CHAPTER 8

Understand me

WEI WEI AND MEI LING

'Before Mum's diagnosis, I thought dementia was just another word for Alzheimer's disease. I'd always heard about people with dementia forgetting their family, losing their memories, and becoming unrecognisable versions of themselves. I was terrified when my mum, Mei Ling, started behaving oddly – getting words muddled, struggling to follow conversations, and becoming unusually fixated on certain ideas. I thought it was only a matter of time before she didn't know who I was.

'It wasn't until we saw a specialist that I learned there are different types of dementia, each with their own symptoms and progression. Mum was diagnosed with frontotemporal dementia (FTD), and while I was still scared, understanding what we were dealing with gave me a strange kind of relief. The doctor explained that FTD tends to affect language and behaviour more than memory, which meant Mum wasn't likely to forget me or our family.

'That knowledge changed everything. Instead of panicking when Mum struggled to find the right words or acted impulsively, I began to see these behaviours as part of her condition rather than something she was doing on purpose. I found ways to make communication easier, like asking simple yes-or-no questions and giving her plenty of time to respond. I also learned that FTD could make her emotions unpredictable, so I stopped taking her outbursts personally.

'It wasn't all plain sailing, I found some of mum's behaviours, like not wanting to throw anything away, difficult to cope with. Having said that, knowing what to expect helped me plan for the future. I

> joined a support group for people who care for someone with FTD, and hearing from others who were walking the same path made me feel less alone. The best part? I could stop dreading the moment Mum might forget me and focus on the time we still had together.
>
> 'We've even found new ways to connect. Mum loves looking through photo albums, and while she can't always describe the memories behind the pictures, she lights up when we flip through them. I've realised that dementia doesn't mean losing everything — it just means finding different ways to hold onto what's most important.'

The aim of this chapter is to outline the different types of dementia to help you to better understand your relative's symptoms. If you know which type of dementia your relative has you can skip over the other types of dementia and just read about the one that is relevant to you and your relative. If you don't know what type of dementia your relative has, contact your GP or the doctor who made the diagnosis. This chapter doesn't shy away from the more challenging symptoms; rather, it arms you with knowledge and practical advice to help you to reduce the incidence of challenging symptoms and deal with those you do encounter with minimal impact on your health and well-being and that of your relative. My aim is for you to be able to connect with your relative and see them as distinct from their symptoms.

The dementia stories and symptom descriptions of the most common forms of dementia outlined below are intended to give a general overview but it is important to remember that these are just a general guide. Your relative may experience only some symptoms, or their symptoms may progress more slowly or more rapidly. If they have mixed dementia their symptoms will, as the name suggests, be a mix of symptoms from several diseases that cause dementia. It can be stressful not knowing what to expect but understanding as much as you can about dementia will help. Section 3 takes a closer look at these symptoms, offering advice and strategies to cope with and manage the more challenging symptoms. You will encounter various health professionals as you journey through dementia. The following box outlines these professions and the roles they will play in your relative's care.

HEALTH PROFESSIONALS

You will be familiar with General Practitioners (GPs) and the role they play in our health. With dementia, consulting your GP is the first port of call. They will assess the situation holistically and may refer you to a specialist for further evaluation. If your relative is diagnosed, the GP will continue managing care, with occasional specialist input as needed.

Specialists

- **Geriatrician:** Focuses on illnesses in older adults, particularly memory and mental decline, often working with a team to support older patients.
- **Neurologist:** Specialises in brain and nervous system disorders; usually for those under 65 with complex conditions.
- **Old age psychiatrist:** An expert in mental health in older people, particularly dementia-related issues.
- **Psychiatrist:** Treats mental health conditions such as depression that may mimic dementia, typically for those under 65.
- **Clinical psychologist:** Assesses memory and cognitive abilities, offering tests and support for those with mental function concerns.
- **Public health nurse:** Provides home visits and coordinates community services, connecting individuals to day care, home care and additional supports like Meals on Wheels or respite care.
- **Social worker:** Offers psychosocial support and advocacy for those with dementia and their families, connecting them to community and hospital services.
- **Occupational therapist:** Helps maintain independence by suggesting home adaptations and equipment for daily activities, such as bathing and mobility.

Dementia is not a disease in and of itself. Rather, it is a term used to describe a collection of symptoms caused by a variety of brain diseases. These diseases damage brain cells in parts of the brain involved in memory, language and learning, resulting in deficits in all three cognitive domains. Unfortunately, to confuse matters, the word dementia is also used as an umbrella term for the neurological conditions that bring about dementia symptoms due to the physical changes they cause in the brain.

Dementia falls under the category of Neurocognitive Disorders (NCDs) rather than being considered a mental illness. The term 'cognitive' refers to mental functions like thinking and memory, while 'neuro' indicates that the symptoms stem from brain disease or a disruption in brain function. NCDs are acquired conditions, meaning they develop during a person's life rather than being present from birth or early childhood. People with NCDs may experience difficulties in areas such as attention, language, learning, memory, planning, social skills, spatial awareness and other cognitive abilities.

NCDs are further classified into two levels: minor and major. Minor NCD, also referred to as Mild Cognitive Impairment (MCI) or prodromal disease (meaning early stage or early warning stage), involves a mild decline in cognitive abilities that doesn't impact the person's independence. A diagnosis of major NCD requires evidence of a noticeable decline in cognitive abilities from a person's earlier levels, based on concerns raised by the individual, a close relative or friend, or a clinician, along with results from formal testing or clinical evaluation. This decline must significantly interfere with the person's ability to live independently. For both minor and major NCDs, the cognitive difficulties should not be due to a mental disorder (like depression or schizophrenia) or appear only when the patient has delirium.

Diagnosis

There are six domains of cognitive function (mental abilities).

1. Complex attention
Your relative may have issues in this domain if they, for example:

- Struggle to follow a book or TV show without getting distracted or forgetting the plot.
- Find it difficult to hold a conversation or make dinner without making mistakes.

- Struggle to focus on a conversation at family functions with multiple conversations going on or in a busy coffee shop with loud music and lots of activity at the counter.
- Are unable to keep up with a fast-paced discussion, needing more time to think before responding, or taking longer to understand and follow instructions.
- Feel confused and agitated in a bustling supermarket with the noise of announcements, conversations and background music, making it hard to concentrate on shopping.

2. Executive functions
Your relative may have issues in this domain if they, for example:

- Struggle to manage both familiar and complex tasks at home or work, such as paying bills or organising a project.
- Need to rely heavily on others to make decisions or plan daily activities such as writing a grocery list or scheduling appointments.
- Have problems grasping abstract concepts – for instance, they might struggle to understand concepts like time (for example, what 'next week' means) or financial matters (such as how interest rates work or why budgeting is important).
- Lack initiative, engaging in tasks only when prompted. They may, for example, need reminders to complete daily routines like brushing their teeth or preparing meals, rather than starting these tasks on their own. Or they may wear the same clothes for days and need prompting to put on fresh clothes.
- Are making poor decisions. For example, they might wear inappropriate clothing for the weather – such as a heavy coat on a hot day – or give away large amounts of money to strangers or through questionable donations.

3. Learning and memory
Your relative may have issues in this domain if they, for example:

- Frequently repeat the same stories or questions within a short time frame.

- Forget items on a shopping list or are unable to remember plans for the day.
- Constantly need reminders to stay focused on tasks.
- Are confused about time and place, not knowing what day, month or season it is or where they are.

4. Language

Your relative may have issues in this domain if they, for example:

- Struggle to find the right words or understand what others are saying, often using vague terms like 'that thing' or 'you know what I mean'.
- Fail to recall the names of close friends or family members.

5. Perceptual-motor function

Your relative may have issues in this domain if they, for example:

- Have significant trouble with activities that were once easy, like using tools, driving, or navigating familiar environments.

6. Social cognition

Your relative may have issues in this domain if they, for example:

- Become insensitive to social norms – for instance, they may interrupt conversations abruptly without noticing it's inappropriate, or they might stand too close to others, invading personal space without realising it, or fail to read social cues such as extending a hand for a handshake.
- Make inappropriate comments – for example, they might comment openly on someone's appearance in a way that seems rude, or bring up private matters in a public setting, unaware of how their words may affect others.
- Laugh inappropriately because they don't fully understand the point of the exchange.
- Avoid social interactions or gatherings – they may, for instance, decline invitations to family events or avoid gatherings with friends, preferring to stay isolated rather than engage socially.

The above criteria relate to a general diagnosis of dementia but, as I mentioned earlier, dementia is a collection of symptoms caused by a variety of different diseases, disorders or conditions. Knowing which type of dementia your relative has will help immensely in navigating the journey as their care partner.

Alzheimer's disease is the most common form of dementia, accounting for 60 to 70 per cent of cases of dementia, so let's begin with that.

Alzheimer's disease

The Alzheimer brain is atrophied compared to a healthy brain and is characterised by cell death and tissue loss. Nobody knows for sure what causes this cell death, but abnormal protein clusters called plaques and twisted strands of another protein, called tangles, are currently the prime suspects. While the majority of people with Alzheimer's disease will have memory complaints, more than one in ten people with the disease have what's referred to as non-amnestic Alzheimer's, where memory function remains unaffected. It can help to think of Alzheimer's disease in three stages.

Early stage

ALICE AND TOM

Alice is 67 and lives with her husband, Tom, who retired 18 months ago. Tom was the breadwinner and Alice gave up work in her twenties when they first married. She stayed at home to raise their family and look after the house. She's a keen baker and loves a game of golf. She also arranges the flowers for her parish church.

Alice had been having what she called 'senior moments' for a couple of years. She'd become a bit absent-minded and was forever losing things about the house. She also had a bit of trouble finding the right word, but she felt that all of this was just a normal part of ageing. After all, she wasn't getting any younger.

When Tom retired, he started to notice that Alice was repeating herself a lot and she also seemed to be struggling to follow conversations. At first, he thought she just wasn't paying attention, but after a bit, when he thought about all of the things that he had noticed together, he felt that something wasn't quite right. With a bit of persuasion, he got Alice to agree to visit their doctor, who sent Alice to the memory clinic for assessment, where she was told she had early-stage Alzheimer's disease.

At this point, Alice's symptoms are really quite mild and she remains independent and manages to do pretty much everything that she was doing before diagnosis. She feels more confident when she sticks to her routine. She is not too keen on trying new things, especially after the incident at the last ladies' golf club outing. Alice always looked forward to their annual outing. Every year, on the longest day, they'd hire a coach and head off for a fancy meal. It was always a great laugh. They went somewhere different every year. Alice's friend Marge says: 'Alice was really enjoying the day when suddenly she came over "all funny" in the restaurant as they were walking back from the bathroom. She became distressed and confused. She looked at me oddly and didn't seem to know where we were or what we were doing there. She became quite frightened and if I'm honest she frightened me too. We calmed her down and eventually she came back to her usual self, but it knocked the stuffing out of her for a bit.'

Alice still bakes a great cake but finds she needs to check her recipe book occasionally and she does find that she gets tired more easily now. She tries to keep positive but some days she feels down and gets frustrated with herself for forgetting things. Tom is great – he keeps the kitchen wall planner up to date and gives Alice gentle reminders if he thinks she might forget a coffee date or dentist appointment, although he did notice she never forgets about a game of golf. Her golf is unaffected, and she still does a great floral display.

In the early stages of Alzheimer's disease, symptoms can be very mild and people with a diagnosis can continue to engage in lots of activities independently. However, they may find some activities challenging and may need to rest more frequently. People in the early stages may:

- Be forgetful.
- Repeat things frequently.
- Struggle to find the right word.
- Find it difficult to follow a conversation.
- Become confused in new places or novel situations.
- Have trouble making decisions or show uncharacteristically poor judgement.
- Have trouble holding interest in other people or activities.
- Avoid trying new things.
- Become withdrawn, depressed, anxious, frustrated or angry.

Mid stage

ALICE AND TOM

Alice remained very independent for about three years. However, her symptoms were gradually getting worse. Tom found himself plugging the gaps a lot more. Five years on from diagnosis and Alice is now 72 and has become much more dependent on Tom, who is the same age. She doesn't sleep well at night and needs help getting dressed and with washing, something that both of them find very tough.

Alice gets very frustrated when she can't do things. Baking has become quite a challenge as she finds the recipes hard to follow, and she struggles with newspapers and TV dramas, especially in the evening when she generally feels tired, a bit crotchety and irritable.

Alice no longer feels confident going out and about on her own as she now gets confused even in familiar places. Thankfully, Marge and her other friends are willing companions, especially as Alice has retained her sense of fun, so she still gets out and about – just not alone and not quite as often as before.

During this middle or moderate stage, the person with Alzheimer's may need your support to carry out everyday activities. This might impact on your relative's self-confidence and they may be upset and withdrawn. They may experience frustration and anger and become argumentative or lose their temper. Common symptoms include:

- Trouble sleeping.
- Difficulty with dressing, washing and meal preparation.
- Forgetting to eat, drink or take medication.
- Finding conversations, TV and reading difficult to follow or confusing.
- Forgetting recent events.
- Getting lost or confused in places that should be familiar.
- Becoming confused about time.
- Restlessness and agitation.
- Believing things are real that are not.

Section 3 gives practical suggestions and strategies to cope with these symptoms and behaviours that can challenge both the person with dementia and their care partner.

Late stage

ALICE AND TOM

Now 76, Alice has advanced dementia and has become quite frail physically and is infection-prone. Some of her friends come to visit but to be honest, the majority don't; they say they find it hard to see Alice this way. Alice enjoys the visits but doesn't always remember who everyone is, although she still knows Tom. She struggles remembering what she had for lunch or even if she had lunch.

Alice eventually developed difficulty swallowing and had a couple of near choking episodes. This really frightened both Tom and Alice. They decided it might be best for her to move into a nursing home where the staff are equipped to deal with this and

> her other increasing nursing needs. Tom spends most of every day there with her, talking to her, holding her hand and listening to old songs together. He didn't have much time for this at home because he was exhausted looking after Alice's fundamental needs such as washing, dressing, food preparation, medications and laundry. Now the nursing home has taken over those activities, he feels they can have more quality time together.

While 'brain things' like memory and language are affected in the early stages of dementia, as the disease progresses and spreads through the brain other functions are impaired. For example, when the brain stem is affected the person with dementia's ability to swallow is compromised. Balance can be impaired, falls become increasingly common and in advanced stages, the ability to maintain upright posture or respond quickly to changes in position may decline. As a consequence of these and other changes in the late stage, the person with Alzheimer's disease will become frail and will need progressively more support, including nursing care. They will find it tough to fight off infection – our immune system can become less effective as we age and is further compromised by dementia pathology – and may become unsteady on their feet, need a wheelchair or be confined to bed. They may have:

- Difficulty recognising people, although there may be flashes of recognition.
- Difficulty eating and/or swallowing.
- Gradual loss of speech or language.
- Incontinence.

Language is only one way we communicate though. Section 3 gives practical tips for communicating, comforting and engaging with your relative at this late stage.

Vascular dementia

Vascular dementia is the second most common form of dementia, accounting for 10 to 20 per cent of cases of dementia. Brain cells are damaged when the blood vessels that supply the brain become narrowed or blocked. This damage can be caused by a stroke, a series of ministrokes or other conditions that affect blood vessels.

OMAR

Omar had a stroke four years ago and was subsequently diagnosed with vascular dementia. He doesn't have memory problems, but he does have sensory issues. He can't drive anymore, which devastated him but was something he just had to accept since he has lost his depth perception. His sensory issues cause him trouble even when he is on foot.

He can't tell where the footpath ends and the road begins anymore. He also struggles with stairs and steps. Everything seems to come at him at once. It's very confusing and scary to be outside. His heart races every time he sees a car because it feels like the car is coming straight at him. The same happens in supermarkets, where people and shopping trollies appear to be coming at him at full tilt.

It's just too stressful for him to go out on his own so he usually has someone with him who keeps reassuring him that he is OK, that nobody is going to crash into him. His companion also has to make sure that Omar doesn't just walk straight out onto the road. For the last four years, Omar's symptoms have been stable. About a month ago, he started having what he calls his 'nothing' moments. He thinks they mainly happen when he is trying to plan or figure something out. He finds these moments scary. He says it's hard to explain but it's as if everything inside his head goes blank. It's very confusing and distressing.

While Alzheimer's disease generally has a gradual progression, vascular dementia can progress in steps. What this means is that symptoms can occur suddenly, for example after a stroke, and remain level for months or years. It is possible for them to remain stable if no other strokes or vascular events occur. Managing health and risk is critical to reduce risk of further strokes and to maintain cognitive stability. However, if the person has another stroke, their symptoms can worsen drastically and remain at that level.

If a series of smaller strokes are the cause of the vascular dementia, then the symptoms can emerge in a more gradual way and may be the consequence of what are referred to as covert strokes. These smaller strokes occur when a small blood vessel in the brain is permanently blocked, causing the brain cells around the area to die. You won't feel a covert stroke as it's happening, but collectively over time multiple smaller strokes chip away at parts of the brain to a point where they impair functioning.

Symptoms can be similar to those found in Alzheimer's disease. People with vascular dementia can be very aware of their condition and sometimes this knowledge can make them more susceptible to depression than people with Alzheimer's disease, who may have less awareness. Changes to personality or emotions don't tend to occur with vascular dementia until later stages. Symptoms may include:

- Memory loss.
- Changes in how the person walks.
- Problems communicating.
- Disorientation.

Then, depending on what area of the brain is affected, other symptoms might include:

- Problems with planning.
- Poor concentration.
- Short periods of confusion.

Dementia with Lewy bodies (DLB)

Lewy bodies are abnormal clumps of protein. The disease is progressive and in the later stages the dementia progresses in a similar way to

Alzheimer's disease. Lewy body demetia accounts for 10 to 15 per cent of dementia cases.

> **CHARLES**
>
> Charles shuffles rather than walks and his head bent forward at the neck makes him seem older than his 75 years. His face is expressionless. He has frequent visual hallucinations and is very clear about, and sometimes terrified by, what he sees. As his dementia has progressed, he has fewer hallucinations. He also has very active dreams, often talking, shouting and thrashing about. As a consequence, he doesn't sleep well at night but nods off a lot during the day. He is often confused but has moments of lucidity, clarity and self-awareness where he is totally present and in possession of his full cognitive faculties.

In the early stages of dementia with Lewy bodies, symptoms can fluctuate dramatically even over the course of a single day. Movement can also be affected, with some symptoms similar to those you might expect in Parkinson's disease, such as tremor, rigidity and slowed movement. Many people with Parkinson's eventually develop dementia. People with DLB may be prone to fainting or falling. This is because dementia with Lewy bodies affects parts of the brain that control things like blood pressure, making them prone to a sudden drop in blood pressure on standing, leading to dizziness and fainting. They can also have hallucinations and prolonged periods of severe confusion. They may sleep during the day but not at night and experience difficulty swallowing.

Approximately 50–80 per cent of people with Parkinson's disease will eventually develop dementia as the disease progresses. This form of dementia is commonly referred to as Parkinson's disease dementia (PDD). The likelihood of developing dementia increases the longer a person has Parkinson's disease. Typically, dementia symptoms may appear about 10–15 years after the initial Parkinson's diagnosis, although this can vary widely. The older a person is when Parkinson's begins and the more severe their physical symptoms, the more likely they are to develop dementia. Cognitive symptoms often include problems with attention, memory, executive function (for example, planning and problem-solving) and visual-spatial skills. Additionally, individuals with Parkinson's disease dementia may experience symptoms such as hallucinations and fluctuations in alertness.

It's worth noting that while Parkinson's disease and dementia with Lewy bodies share some overlapping features, they are considered distinct conditions. In dementia with Lewy bodies, cognitive symptoms typically appear before or at the same time as motor symptoms, while in Parkinson's disease dementia, cognitive symptoms usually emerge after several years of motor symptoms.

Frontotemporal dementia (FTD)

As the name suggests, this form of dementia is caused by brain cells degenerating (breaking down) in the frontal and temporal lobes of the brain. The frontal lobes play a key role in personality and many behaviours, including social and sexual behaviour. The temporal lobes are involved in understanding and producing language. FTD accounts for somewhere between 5 and 10 per cent of cases of dementia.

> **LILLY**
>
> Lilly's dementia makes her very disinhibited. This means she has no filter. She simply says what she sees and thinks. She just ploughs right in there with both feet. If she is on the bus, she can't stop herself from commenting on people's clothes or weight. She will even say things of a sexual nature, things that belong only inside her head.
>
> The other day she told the girl behind the cold meats counter that her acne was enough to put anyone off their food and she should be working in the back storeroom, not on a counter serving food people have to eat. People assume she's wilfully rude or mad, but worst of all is when they think she is just looking to start a fight.

> Her family are concerned about her safety and got her some cards printed that explain she has FTD. They try to go with her when she goes out if they can, but she doesn't always want that and it's tough for them as they have jobs and lives of their own.
>
> Her FTD killed her marriage. It took a while for a proper diagnosis and her husband left because he couldn't cope with what he called her 'antics'. They'd been apart for a while by the time she was diagnosed. She says she doesn't care – well, she does but she doesn't. She says it's hard to explain. One of the symptoms of her dementia is apathy so she finds it hard to care. She could talk about herself all day but can't be bothered to ask other people how they are.
>
> Her family understand that she has no control over what she says. But they are human and sometimes what she says is hard for them to take. Once she starts on a rant she can't stop and can say some really personal, hurtful things. She also has huge difficulty making decisions and has really poor judgement, which hasn't helped her situation.

Early symptoms of frontotemporal dementia will vary depending on which part of the brain is affected. If the temporal lobes are affected, symptoms will relate to language. If the frontal lobes are affected, the person will have problems with planning, organisation, motivation, controlling their emotions and maintaining socially appropriate behaviour and can include:

- Problems speaking to or understanding others.
- Personality change.
- Change in eating patterns.
- Lack of social awareness – they may say or do socially inappropriate things.
- Lack of personal awareness – they may fail to take care of personal hygiene.

Mixed dementia

The older people are when they get dementia, the more likely they will be given a diagnosis of mixed dementia. This simply means that they have a combination of Alzheimer's disease, vascular dementia and dementia with Lewy bodies.

> ### ZARA AND NIA
>
> Nia had mixed dementia. She had a variety of symptoms, a few from this type and a couple from that – like many older people, her dementia was of the Heinz 57 variety. Nia could ask the same question repeatedly but she never for a moment forgot who her daughter, Zara, was. With time, she lost a lot of words, but Zara, a psychology lecturer, still managed to understand her, and she certainly always seemed able to understand Zara.
>
> Nia had hallucinations. For the most part these were very pleasant, and she often laughed at them and pointed to the little people dancing on the wall at the other side of the room. Occasionally, she pointed to people's faces on the street because they were missing bits or had facial features in the wrong places. That did seem to upset her and make her turn away.
>
> Zara explained to Nia that her brain was creating pictures that weren't actually there. Zara encouraged Nia to talk about them because she enjoyed hearing Nia describe what she saw. Just saying this removed a huge amount of anxiety and stress for Nia and Zara genuinely did enjoy hearing her descriptions of what she saw. Nia found some comfort in that.
>
> She was also frequently depressed and had a number of psychotic episodes, but these were often brought on by severe urinary tract infections. After these episodes, she seemed to have a somewhat vague awareness that she had behaved in a way that was out of character or that she felt uncomfortable about. Nia could be quite

> 'frontal' at times, saying what she thought and using expletives that Zara didn't even know she knew. At other times, Nia was very aware that she wasn't quite herself and could be very controlled about what she said and did. She became prone to infection and spent a good deal of time in hospital. Over time, she became very frail and had terrible difficulty swallowing. Eventually, she even had to have food thickener put into a glass of water or a cup of tea to prevent further choking episodes that required the Heimlich manoeuvre.

Young/early-onset dementia

When dementia symptoms appear before the age of 65 it is referred to as early-onset dementia or young/er-onset dementia. Both late/er-onset dementia and young/er-onset dementia are caused by a range of different diseases. However, a wider range of diseases causes young-onset dementia and those affected are more likely to have a rarer form of dementia. People with young-onset dementia are more likely to have problems with movement, walking and balance. Memory loss is not usually an early symptom. Because of the patient's age and the presentation of symptoms, young-onset dementia is often misdiagnosed.

Alzheimer's disease is the most common type of young-onset dementia. Younger people with Alzheimer's disease are much more likely to have an unusual form and their initial symptoms will differ depending on the form they have. For example, problems reading, figuring out visual information, or judging distances are early symptoms of posterior cortical atrophy (PCA), while difficulties with language, such as word-finding are often the first symptoms to manifest in logopenic aphasia. Issues with making decisions, planning and behaving inappropriately in social situations are early symptoms of dysexecutive Alzheimer's disease.

The earlier symptoms start the more likely there is a genetic cause. Familial Alzheimer's disease usually starts in 30s, 40s or 50s and is caused by a genetic mutation that runs in families. It is a very rare form of the disease but highly heritable with a 50% chance that a parent will pass the disease mutation on to their children.

People with Down's syndrome and some other learning disabilities have an increased risk of developing dementia at a young age. Alzheimer's disease is the most common cause of dementia in people with Down's syndrome.

Frontotemporal dementia discussed earlier in this chapter is also more common in younger people with dementia than in older people and is usually diagnosed between the ages of 45 and 65.

Vascular dementia is closely linked to diabetes and stroke and so can also be the cause of dementia in people under 65.

If you are caring for a relative with young onset dementia your circumstances will be considerably different to those of a person caring for someone with late/er onset dementia; you may be coping with raising young children while also providing care for your spouse. Your relative may have trouble continuing to work and may lose their income but not yet be in receipt of a pension. It is really important that you seek support from sources that understand your unique needs and those of your relative. A good place to start is with the diagnosing professional or your GP.

While it is important to understand dementia, I am very conscious that reading about these symptoms can be rather depressing. The next chapter is much more uplifting, I promise, and indeed section 3 in its entirety is about practical ways to make life better despite dreadful symptoms that become part of everyday life.

Section 2: Summary

Key messages

- It is easy to be fooled by dementia into thinking your relative is no longer there.
- Your relative is still a person with feelings, needs, dreams and desires.
- The person with dementia is an adult and deserves to be treated as such.
- Your relative is still your parent, sibling or spouse, reflect this in your interactions.
- Your relative may no longer be able to articulate what they are experiencing but they will be aware that you are treating them differently or like a child.
- Patience is a skill rather than a trait – it can be learned.
- Doing nothing is boring, accelerates decline and diminishes independence.
- Don't underestimate the power of human touch.
- Your role as care partner is not to decide for them but rather to support them to exercise their right to decide, whether you agree with their decision or not. Involve your relative in all decisions – 'nothing about you without you.'
- Treat your relative with dignity and respect.
- Seeking respite care or professional help is not a sign of failure but a proactive step in ensuring the best care for your relative while maintaining your own health.
- In the initial period following diagnosis your relative may deny diagnosis and minimise symptoms. This is a common defence mechanism, so don't force your relative to acknowledge their diagnosis.
- Dementia is caused by a number of brain diseases.
- Symptoms will vary depending on the specific condition.
- Everyone's experience of dementia is unique.

Practical tips

- Speak to your relative as an equal and use grown-up words.
- Make sure that everyone involved with your relative's care:
  - treats your relative with dignity and respect as an adult.
  - uses terminology that is familiar to your relative.
  - is aware of your relative's preferences, likes and dislikes.
- Cultivate patience and find the good in the situation.
- Adjust your expectations to account for your relative's dementia.
- Find the good in difficult situations. Consciously switch your focus from unpleasant triggers to something more pleasant.
- Inject a little humour – try to lighten how you view the situation.
- Empower your relative to be as independent as possible. Support them to contribute to their own life. Do with, not for. Consider how you might partner your relative on tasks rather than take over completely.
- Your relative remains capable of becoming bored; remember to provide opportunities for them to engage with life in a meaningful way.
- As the disease progresses and the usual means of communication are no longer possible, become observant and watch out for more subtle means of communication such as a furrowed brow, a wince or a hint of a smile.
- Stimulate your relative's senses through scent and touch especially if their sight and vision are failing.
- Involve them in as many decisions as possible. Even little things like giving them a choice of what to eat or what to wear each day can restore a sense of control to their lives.
- Always assume your relative can make their own decisions unless proven otherwise – this applies to everyday decisions like what to wear or what to eat.
- If you are unsure about the right course of action in complex situations, consulting with a social worker, an older persons' advocacy group, a solicitor familiar with elder care or the Alzheimer's Association can provide clarity and direction.
- Balance risks with rights.

- Avoid being overprotective and paternalistic. Make adjustments to room layouts for maximum safety. Night lights, removal of trip hazards and carefully placed furniture can minimise the risk of falls.
- Provide a safe place for your relative to walk. If you have a garden remove trip hazards, and provide seating and use lights, ornaments and scented plants to make an interesting place to stop and linger. If you don't have a garden add a walk in a local green space to your daily routine.
- Some councils have a Neighbourhood Return Scheme where local residents guide people with dementia back home. Contact your local council; if one doesn't exist ask them to start one. Have discrete conversations with local businesses asking them to keep an eye out for your relative. Most people are more than happy to help.
- Pop notes into the pockets of your relative's clothing with your contact details.
- Ask medical professionals what type of dementia your relative has.
- Familiarise yourself with the symptoms and trajectory of their specific type of dementia – you don't need to learn about all types.

SECTION 3
Live Well

Considerable work has been carried out by researchers, health professionals and people living with dementia themselves to identify ways to adapt, manage difficulties and live a good life with dementia. None of the activities, strategies or interventions outlined in this section will cure dementia but they have been shown to delay the onset of symptoms, change the trajectory of the disease, improve day-to-day functioning, boost health and well-being, increase social participation and enhance overall quality of life. People in the early and middle stages of dementia, reliable reporters of their own quality of life, consistently say mood, involvement in pleasant activities and the ability to perform the everyday tasks of daily living are the key factors that influence their quality of life. Care partners feel that mood, engagement in pleasant activities, as well as physical and cognitive functioning, are important for their relative's quality of life.

Recent research into the priorities and preferences of people living with dementia, which combined findings from multiple studies carried out between 1990 and 2019, found that the majority of people with dementia and their spouses demonstrated altruistic preferences – that is, they each put the other's needs before their own. The majority of people with dementia with the capacity to do so ranked their care partner's quality of life as their highest priority and vice versa. It's helpful to remind yourself regularly that your relative most likely wants you to have a good quality of life. This section of the book aims to help both you and your relative to fulfil that need to look after each other – and to live well with dementia.

When it comes to understanding what makes treatments effective for people living with dementia, research with both individuals and their care partners highlights several main goals. These include better cognitive function, improved ability to carry out daily tasks, fewer behavioural issues, slower decline, and an overall better quality of life. Section 3 deals with each of these in turn. Chapter 10, 'Making the most of what you've got', covers evidence-based interventions and therapies developed to improve cognitive function and day-to-day functional ability. Chapter 11, 'Minimising the tough stuff', focuses on improving your understanding and management of psychiatric symptoms and challenging behaviours. Chapter 12, 'Maximising the good stuff', focuses on ways to improve quality of life and delay onset of symptoms.

CHAPTER 9

Making the most of what you've got

> ### JOHN AND ANNE
>
> 'People tend to catastrophise the situation when given a diagnosis, but my Anne was the exact same person as the day before. We never discussed the diagnosis but continued our life and adapted as Anne's memory deteriorated. She suffered from osteoporosis so in time she needed a walking stick, then a stroller, and finally a wheelchair. A diagnosis of early-onset dementia can be devastating, but my advice is take one day at a time.
>
> 'In the early days, they may get angry and aggressive. This is understandable. They know they are slowly changing because of memory loss. They use a lot of energy covering it up and coping. Each day they wake up and have to reboot. Who am I? Where am I? What have I to do today?
>
> 'People ask, how is Anne? The professional asks, how are you? They know if you get ill or depressed, the 'whole ship' sinks. Take all the help you can get and ask for more. I was very worried the first time Anne had to be in hospital (she couldn't find her way around the house). A young woman was appointed to take care of Anne. I was reluctant to use respite but I found that Anne was re-energised when she went to respite, mainly because of all the social interaction she had.
>
> 'The way to a good life and health is the same for us all: exercise, diet and social interaction. Loneliness is the hidden symptom. Friends disappear, they don't know how to deal with it or interact.

> They should just act normal and preferably call in pairs. Anne's personality was there to the end – as one person put it, 'her essence'. During COVID, when we had to cocoon, we saw little difference, that had been our life. I always say dementia is not contagious. I never tried to hide that Anne had dementia, I would introduce her and then introduce myself as her memory. Anne was happy with that.'

Researchers who combined the results of multiple studies carried out over a 29-year period reported that when people with dementia are asked, they say they do not want to be a burden, they want a good quality of life, they want to do as much for themselves as possible, they want to have confidence in their own ability to accomplish daily tasks and they want to have fun and experience pleasure. Essentially, they want to make the most of what they've got.

In the early stages of the disease, people with dementia not only retain cognitive and functional abilities but can also be capable of learning new things. Despite having the disease, the brain of a person with dementia retains the ability to change and can recruit additional neural networks to compensate for the damage caused by disease. This means that, with the right support, people in the early stages of the disease should be able to harness their retained abilities to better manage daily activities, continue to enjoy life and participate in society.

Programmes designed to help people with dementia and their care partners enjoy a better quality of life usually focus on two main areas. Some programmes aim to improve memory and thinking skills. Others help people adapt to the challenges of daily activities so they can live as independently as possible, despite any difficulties with memory or thinking. For example, cognitive training and stimulation therapies work on boosting thinking skills directly. On the other hand, cognitive rehabilitation, sometimes known as neuropsychological rehabilitation, helps people find ways to manage daily tasks more effectively, taking into account the challenges brought on by dementia.

Brain training, also known as cognitive training, is designed to improve specific mental abilities such as attention or memory through exercises that are repeated regularly. You might have seen apps marketed to older adults promising to enhance brain function. However, experts generally agree that these types of exercises don't lead to real-life benefits. Despite some claims, there's no solid evidence that brain training can improve everyday functioning or make daily tasks easier for older adults with mild cognitive issues or those in the early stages of dementia. Research analysing multiple studies has found that these exercises do not have a measurable impact on daily life or overall mental ability.

In contrast, there is considerable evidence for the clinical effectiveness of Cognitive Stimulation Therapy (CST), a group-based treatment designed to boost cognitive and social skills among people with mild to moderate dementia, discussed in this chapter. It has been found to improve memory and thinking skills in people with mild to moderate dementia and quality of life in those who completed group CST. It is important to stimulate cognitive function in the mild to moderate stages of dementia to preserve functioning for as long as possible. Without mental stimulation, decline in cognitive abilities can happen faster.

CST is widely available in the UK and is recognised as an effective non-pharmacological treatment for people with mild to moderate dementia. The National Health Service (NHS) supports and sometimes offers CST as part of the care services for dementia patients, recognising its benefits in improving cognitive function and enhancing quality of life.

CST sessions in the UK are usually provided through memory clinics, community centres and sometimes in care homes, typically involving structured group activities designed to stimulate thinking and memory. These activities are often enjoyable and aim to engage patients socially, which also helps to combat isolation and depression, common issues among those with dementia.

If you are interested in CST for yourself or a loved one, you can speak to your GP or a memory service provider in your area. They can provide more detailed information on availability and referrals. Additionally, some local Alzheimer's Society branches, as well as other dementia support organisations, may offer or be able to direct you to available CST programmes.

These interventions are most beneficial when started early on. Early cognitive interventions help the individual make the most of what they've got by building on aspects of memory that are preserved and by developing ways to compensate for other cognitive impairments, which can help to maintain or even enhance function and lessen disability.

Cognitive rehabilitation acknowledges that the challenges faced by a person with dementia aren't all due to the disease in their brain – other things like losing confidence, being afraid to fail or feeling anxious can impact significantly on the person's quality of life. This approach acknowledges that other factors in the person's life, social circles or surroundings can disable the individual. Understanding this is important because addressing these non-disease factors can reduce disability and improve quality of life.

Cognitive stimulation

Cognitive stimulation therapy (CST) is an evidence-based, structured therapy specifically developed for the cognitive symptoms of dementia. It is widely used in the UK and available in 39 countries. The therapy aims to engage the person with dementia in enjoyable activities in a group setting. Typically, a small group (6–12) of people with dementia meet for 45 minutes, twice a week, for 14 weeks to enjoy a variety of games and activities that stimulate thinking, language skills, concentration and memory. Ideally, people with dementia need to participate in a variety of activities to stimulate different cognitive areas. Evidence suggests that CST produces benefits equivalent to a six-month delay in the expected cognitive decline in people with mild to moderate dementia. More specific benefits reported include improvements in communication and social interaction, quality of life, mood and depression plus reduced 'caregiver burden' and minimisation of aggression and other behaviours that challenge. More generally, attending sessions can give your relative a sense of purpose, build self-esteem and confidence and offer opportunities to socialise and to share their experiences with others. Activities might include music, creative activities, puzzles, word games and discussions of topics of relevance or interest.

Some groups incorporate physical exercise, which improves blood flow to the brain and triggers the release of a chemical called brain-derived neurotrophic factor (BDNF). This chemical makes it easier for the brain to adapt and change and grow new connections between brain cells. CST has also been delivered on a one-to-one basis but there is little research available on how effective that is.

Cognitive rehabilitation

Cognitive rehabilitation and CST have different goals. Cognitive stimulation focuses on cognitive function, specific cognitive areas or overall cognitive functioning. Cognitive rehabilitation focuses on the practical and aims to make everyday life easier for people living with mild to moderate dementia by helping them adapt to some of the changes that dementia can bring. It can be used to help people to find ways around issues with, for example, concentration, memory and language. Cognitive rehabilitation is generally delivered by a trained healthcare professional such as a clinical psychologist, occupational therapist or nurse, who will help your relative to understand how to use these strategies. It is then up to the individual with dementia, with the support of their care partner, to practise and implement the strategies between sessions. Understanding the strategies used in cognitive rehabilitation will help you to support your relative between sessions.

> 'I had terrible trouble remembering important numbers such as the pin codes for my bank card and my phone and the registration of my car. I'd also stopped playing darts because I struggled to remember my friends' names. I'd stopped using cash as I got muddled and I worried I'd lose it. That meant I couldn't buy drinks when we played darts because I had no cash and I couldn't recall the pin for my card.' – George

In a few short sentences, George illustrates the devastating impact that seemingly small issues like forgetting names, pins and other codes can have on the quality and enjoyment of life. Even more worrying is the fact that George and many others like him cope with these issues by withdrawing from life. His fear of embarrassment is so big that George would rather deprive himself of life's pleasures by avoiding social situations. Consequently, he unwittingly risks accelerating the progression of the disease through disuse and lack of social and mental stimulation.

Cognitive rehabilitation is a personalised therapy that helps people with cognitive impairments to improve their daily lives. It uses a problem-solving approach to address the challenges caused by these impairments. The main goal of this therapy is to help individuals function as well as possible despite their cognitive difficulties, helping them manage everyday tasks, engage in meaningful activities and maintain their independence.

Cognitive rehabilitation focuses on what matters most to each person, helping them feel in control of their lives and retain a sense of who they are. This approach takes into account each individual's unique experiences, motivations, values, preferences, skills and needs, as well as their relationships and surroundings. Unlike therapies that try to directly improve cognitive skills, cognitive rehabilitation offers practical solutions to manage the everyday challenges that come with cognitive impairment.

This therapy aims to build confidence by working on personal goals that truly matter to the individual, making a real difference in their daily life. It's a personalised, problem-solving approach that empowers people with dementia to engage in and manage their everyday activities. Cognitive rehabilitation recognises that each person's life experiences, values and motivations make them unique, and it uses this holistic perspective to enhance their independence, functioning and social involvement.

Sometimes called cognitive reablement, this therapy isn't about 'fixing' or restoring cognitive function. Instead, it's a solutions-focused approach that tackles the specific impacts of cognitive impairments on daily life, such as the challenges George might face.

The process involves setting personal goals and identifying areas where the person with dementia wants to improve. Because dementia can make it hard to apply new skills in different situations, cognitive rehabilitation works directly within the context where those skills will be used, making it easier for individuals to adopt strategies that suit their own lives. If your relative's cognitive impairments have already progressed to the point where they interfere with their ability to understand or engage in the process, a practitioner can help you to use effective strategies to support and enable your relative.

The process usually begins with the person with dementia working with a trained therapist to identify meaningful goals that are important to them. They will practise a few different strategies and then decide on their preferred approach. You will then work with your relative to practise the preferred strategies until they feel confident using them.

GEORGE

'I told my therapist that I would love to be able to remember the pins for my phone and my credit card, my car registration and the names of my darts buddies. I worked with my therapist on each of the numbers one at a time. Once we felt confident that I had learned the number, we moved on to the next one. I learned about chunking numbers. Instead of trying to remember four digits 1 – 5 – 0 – 6, I focused on learning just one number, 1,506. I also learned to use a mnemonic system where I associated each number with a specific location, so for my car registration, I visualised the different numbers and letters in specific locations in my car, for example: in the glove box, on the steering wheel, on the gear stick and so on.

'To remember the names of my darts buddies, we used photos and worked on one name at a time. My therapist showed me the photo, we discussed the photo and the name. We generated associations that I could use to assist recall – for example, smiley Simon has a gold filling in one of his front teeth. Working through each of the five names I wanted to remember, we identified a visual association or a stand-out story about the person, linking it to the name – Liam likes the ladies (he's a real charmer). I really had to work hard with the therapist at each session and with my wife every day between sessions to get to the point where I could

> recall as I needed to. The therapist had a very specific, research-based approach which has been shown to work. For the name remembering it went something like this: first the therapist would present me with hints and cues to try to spark my memory, then she would present the same prompts in reverse order to see if I could recall them. I would practise and repeat this. Then the therapist would test my recall after increasing intervals – 30 seconds, 1 minute, 2 minutes, 5 minutes, and 10 minutes. If I couldn't recall the mnemonics and the name, we repeated it until I was able to reliably recall it after 10 minutes. It was hard work, but the sense of achievement was great. My wife, Maisie, was brilliant helping me and nudging me to practise if I got lazy. Her help and support were critical. I'm so glad that I persevered. I'm back playing darts, which has made a huge difference to my mood and my life. I can also reliably remember the pin for my phone and for my credit card. It is definitely worth the effort.'

Goal-setting

Goal-setting is an important aspect of cognitive rehabilitation and something that you can work on with your relative.

Having goals enriches life, giving it purpose and meaning. This is something that applies to all of us, including those living with dementia and their care partners. Following diagnosis, it is easy to fall into the trap of seeing only dementia in the future. The disease can loom so large that it can blind us to other, brighter possibilities. Working towards specific meaningful goals can have a positive impact, shifting focus away from the disease to a future where joy and pleasure can be had.

The cognitive rehabilitation practitioner will work with your relative and with you to figure out where difficulties occur and help come up with a plan, with goals that meet the needs and desires of you both. They can then help identify changes that need to be made to help improve your relative's independence and day-to-day skills and everyday abilities. This could be anything from preparing dinner to using smart technology, going to the local Men's Shed, establishing local landmarks to avoid getting lost, to playing games with grandchildren. As a care partner you can also encourage and support your relative to set specific goals that will help them feel more confident and in control of their lives. It's also important that you don't give up on your own future, so do use the ideas in this section to help you to think about your own goals as well as those of your relative. Goals reflect our desires, our dreams, our wishes. You may feel that many of those have been shattered by the diagnosis. This section will help you to revisit that viewpoint.

Successful goals tend to be *SMART:* Specific – Measurable – Achievable – Relevant – Time-bound. For example:

Goal: Introduce a simple tool to improve memory for daily routines.

Specific: Your relative will use a daily planner to write down three key activities each morning.

Measurable: Success will be measured by their ability to remember and complete at least two of the three planned activities daily.

Achievable: You will help your relative to choose realistic tasks and make it easy for your relative to record them – for example, by writing prompts in the planner and by keeping it in a prominent place close to a clock and a calendar.

Relevant: This goal supports independence and enhances memory recall, which are things your relative wants to improve.

Time-bound: The person will practise this goal for two weeks, with weekly check-ins to assess progress.

Goal: Increase social interaction to reduce feelings of isolation before winter comes.

Specific: Your relative will engage in a ten-minute conversation with a family member or friend every day.

Measurable: Success will be tracked by documenting each conversation.

Achievable: Conversations can happen in person, over the phone, or via video calls to accommodate different circumstances.

Relevant: This goal addresses social engagement, which can improve mood and cognitive stimulation.

Time-bound: The goal will be revisited after one month to evaluate impact and adjust as necessary.

AMY AND NIALL

Amy provides care for Niall, her husband of 51 years. Her goal was to have some 'me time', preferably an outdoor activity that involved doing something with tangible results.

'I decided to cultivate a small garden just outside the sunroom where my husband Niall liked to nap in the afternoon. The location of the garden allowed me to ensure that Niall remained safe while I did something rewarding and gained a sense of achievement and purpose independent of my caregiving role. My goal to create a garden to provide me with a tranquil space and a source of fresh herbs and flowers was specific. I kept the garden small and manageable. I focused on easy-to-care-for plants that bring me joy and that I can use in my cooking or for decorative purposes. My objective was to have at least five different types of plants thriving in my wee garden. I tracked my progress by taking photos every week to document the growth of my plants and by keeping a simple journal of my gardening activities. Considering my responsibilities and physical capabilities, I opted for a reasonably sized raised-bed garden, which I found easier to maintain once my son built the frame. I started with seedlings rather than seeds to see results more quickly and ensure the task was manageable.'

Gardening provides Amy with a personal ongoing project that boosts her sense of well-being and independence, offering a creative outlet and physical activity. It's a meaningful distraction that enriches her life and brings her personal satisfaction outside of her caregiving duties. At the outset she set a goal to have her garden established within two months. This gave her enough time to plan, prepare and see the initial results of her efforts without feeling rushed. This goal is tailored to give her something positive to focus on, promoting a sense of achievement and purpose while improving her quality of life through engaging with nature, enhancing her living environment and providing a peaceful retreat while still carrying out her caregiving responsibilities.

This section will also help you to help your relative to identify simple changes that could make a big difference, not just in terms of improving functionality, but also in terms of mood, well-being and self-confidence. Your role as care partner is to support and enable progress and celebrate successes with your relative.

It is important to keep goals simple and specific. It is also essential to focus on things that can be changed. Small wins accumulate and can add up to big changes in mood and quality of life. The following probing questions and prompts can help you and your relative to identify goals that matter to both of you.

- How do you feel about your dementia?
- How does it affect you day-to-day?
- What is one thing that has changed with your dementia diagnosis that you would like to work on (e.g. remembering names, cooking, using the phone or TV remote, playing poker, socialising).
- What small change could make a meaningful difference for you?
- What would you like to start doing?
- Is there a hobby or interest that you would like to pursue?
- Would you like to spend more time with friends?
- Would you like to manage things around the house better?

In the first instance, the therapist will assess your relative's cognitive capacity, functional ability, their current needs and their strengths, taking account of relationships, emotions and environment. This phase allows the therapist to identify your relative's potential and highlight activities where your relative is functioning below their capacity. For example, George's loss of confidence and fear of embarrassment has resulted in his reluctance to engage in activities that he enjoys. The consequent loss of skills creates unnecessary burden and excess disability. Depending on what emerges from this information-gathering phase, the therapist may first address issues such as lack of confidence, depression and anxiety.

Many people with dementia experience low mood and apathy, which may need to be addressed at the start of therapy. Behavioural activation (using behaviour to influence mood) is used to encourage engagement in activities that are usually enjoyable. The feelings of engagement and pleasure experienced can then motivate the individual to make positive change. Starting the cognitive rehabilitation process can be daunting and can result in fear, frustration or despair. In this case, the therapists are trained to provide vital psychological support to acknowledge these emotions and help individuals develop ways to manage and overcome these potential barriers to successfully attaining their goals.

Working with your therapist, you and your relative can identify activities that are important to them and that they would like to work on. The therapist uses this information, along with an understanding of your relative's cognitive abilities, skills, support and environment, to decide what kind of progress is realistic. By understanding these challenges, you can work together to find solutions that help your relative reach their goals – whether by practising certain skills, using memory aids or managing emotions.

The therapist will choose the most effective approach from a variety of tools and strategies. These might include modifying activities or the environment, learning new ways to approach tasks, adapting old habits, using compensatory techniques or incorporating assistive technology. Once a solution is selected, a plan is created and put into action.

For example, if your relative struggles to prepare meals safely, you might simplify the kitchen layout, removing unnecessary items and placing frequently used items in easy-to-reach spots. Additionally, using clear labels on cabinets can make it easier for them to find what they need.

If managing medication is a challenge for your relative, the therapist might work with them to establish a new routine, such as taking medicine immediately after breakfast, to create a consistent and easily remembered association.

If your relative was used to driving but is now having difficulty, adapting the habit could mean learning to use public transport or asking for help with transport. The therapist may focus on gradually building comfort with these alternatives.

If memory issues make it hard for your relative to remember daily tasks, using a whiteboard or a visual checklist in a prominent place (for example, the fridge) can act as a reminder for essential activities like eating meals or taking medication.

If your relative is prone to getting disorientated outside, a smartphone app could be used to help them find their way home or to alert you if they feel lost.

Once a solution is chosen, the therapist creates a step-by-step plan to integrate these strategies into daily life, adjusting as needed to ensure they're effective and sustainable.

Progress towards therapy goals is regularly reviewed and adjusted as needed. Throughout this journey, the therapist provides psychological support and encourages a positive, problem-solving mindset. Cognitive rehabilitation focuses on practical problem-solving and setting goals, often drawing on other behavioural therapy methods.

The ultimate aim of cognitive rehabilitation is to make a meaningful difference in daily life. It's essential that the skills learned translate into real-world benefits and can be applied to similar situations. To ensure this, interventions are often carried out in real-life settings where these skills will be used.

Where possible, carers and family members are included to support these changes in day-to-day life. Cognitive rehabilitation is a collaborative effort, and carers play a key role. This therapy also recognises the needs of carers, offering psychological support and connecting them with additional resources. The therapist will work to balance the needs of both the person with dementia and their care partner, acknowledging that this can sometimes be challenging to achieve.

Cognitive rehabilitation is most successful when led by a trained therapist. Accessing a cognitive rehabilitation therapist in the UK depends on several factors, including where you live, your specific needs and whether you are seeking services through the NHS or privately. Cognitive rehabilitation therapy (CRT) is sometimes available through the NHS, particularly for people recovering from stroke, brain injury or certain neurological conditions. For people with dementia, however, access may be more limited and varies by region. Accessing cognitive rehabilitation on the NHS typically requires a referral from a GP or specialist. This process may involve long waiting times, as demand often exceeds availability. Services depend on local NHS trusts, which means some areas may have dedicated cognitive rehabilitation therapists while others do not.

Cognitive rehabilitation therapists are available privately, but this can be costly, and fees vary widely depending on the therapist's experience and location. Private therapy may be more accessible in terms of waiting times and flexibility. Organisations like the British Psychological Society (BPS), the Royal College of Occupational Therapists (RCOT) and the British Neuropsychological Society (BNS) provide directories of qualified professionals. Some charities, like the Alzheimer's Society, Headway and Dementia UK, may offer or connect people with cognitive support services, including cognitive rehabilitation, or have resources and support workers trained in cognitive strategies. Local councils may offer assessments and some support services through adult social care. If a person with dementia is eligible, social services can sometimes arrange support that includes elements of cognitive rehabilitation. Cognitive rehabilitation is still an emerging field, particularly for conditions like dementia, so even when services exist, they may not be widely promoted or easy to find.

If this therapy doesn't feel like a good fit for you, or you are unable to access a therapist, you and your relative can always work together to create a plan yourselves to achieve your own goals. Having a specific goal gives life purpose and meaning and makes us feel more confident and in control of our lives and our future. Goals don't have to be big or dramatic. To be honest, it's probably better to stick to small, attainable goals. Take things one step at a time. Small wins will still activate the reward and pleasure centres in your brain, making you more motivated to achieve your next small goal. Small goals soon add up to life-changing victories. Take one day at a time and break down your plan of action into small steps. Be realistic about what you or your relative can achieve, accept that some things cannot be changed and focus your attention on those that can.

Helen

Helen Rochford-Brennan was diagnosed with young-onset dementia at 61 in 2011. She felt utter despair on diagnosis. She resigned from her high-powered job and stopped her volunteer work. She was unable to speak about her diagnosis and entered a very dark place until a health professional suggested that she volunteer for research. She contacted the university where I worked. Her timing was perfect. We were looking for volunteers for a research project about a cognitive rehabilitation intervention for people living with dementia at the precise time Helen made contact. Taking part in our research study changed her life. She has spoken since about how cognitive rehabilitation gave her the confidence to speak openly about her diagnosis. Helen and I have become friends and to this day she amazes and inspires me with what she has achieved while living with dementia. On moving from despair to being a pioneer in dementia advocacy, she says she has gone from 'worrier to warrior'. In 2018 she was awarded an honorary degree from the National University of Ireland (Galway). Helen adopts a human-rights approach as she campaigns to raise awareness of dementia, speaking at international conferences, contributing to committees and think-tanks and giving media interviews. Her disease continues to progress but with appropriate strategies and the support of her loyal and ever-present friend, supporter and travel companion Carmel Geoghegan, she continues to campaign. On living with dementia, she says: 'It's a different life, but it's still a good life. Don't be afraid to say you have a problem,' she says. 'Just because I have a cognitive impairment doesn't mean I can't function. I've gone from thinking my life was over, to a place that I could never have dreamed of. Because of Alzheimer's, I've addressed royalty, governments, the European Parliament, world health organisations and global pharma companies. My message is this: "Please do not lose your voice to dementia."'

CHAPTER 10

Minimising the tough stuff

> **MAINTAINING A LIFE OUTSIDE CARING**
>
> **John**
> 'You both still have a life to lead. In the early stage the person behaves as normal. In the middle stage they need more help, dressing, eating, etc. The last stage can be very difficult. Fortunately, Anne passed away before she reached the late stage. But you have done your best so no regrets. It's vital that you maintain some outside activities, because when you resume normal life – you have a life.'

While changes in cognitive functioning are the main criteria for a diagnosis of dementia, behavioural and psychological symptoms in dementia (BPSD), also known as neuropsychiatric symptoms, are common and often cause the most stress and burden. Coping with the kind of behavioural changes that can occur as the disease progresses can be incredibly tough, especially if those behaviours are completely out of character or involve aggression, delusions or hallucinations. Neuropsychiatric symptoms can be upsetting and physically and mentally exhausting and based on research could rapidly push you into crisis. The presence of behavioural and psychological symptoms increases the burden for you. If your relative is affected, you may experience increased caregiving demands and responsibilities; some behaviours may mean that your relative needs constant supervision and support. Dealing with these types of symptoms can be disruptive and leave you feeling frustrated, helpless, burnt out or sad. The behaviours can add to stress and make it difficult for you to engage in self-care. They can also restrict your social activities, limiting your access to support and increasing feelings of isolation. This chapter aims to help you understand these behaviours and offer some positive coping strategies and practical advice on how to respond in adaptive ways that will help to ease the tensions that can arise.

I am very conscious that the descriptions of symptoms in this chapter may be frightening, especially if you are reading this soon after diagnosis or in the early stages of the disease. Your relative may only occasionally experience neuropsychiatric symptoms or their symptoms may be mild or relatively easy to manage. You might find it useful to read the general advice in the early part of the chapter rather than reading about all the possible neuropsychiatric symptoms. Then consider the remainder of the chapter a guide to help you to identify or manage symptoms that you can dip in and out of if you are concerned about changes in your relative's behaviour.

> **KEEPING YOU AND YOUR RELATIVE SAFE**
>
> If your relative is showing signs of agitation or aggression (see more on page 212) and is likely to put you or themselves at risk then it is best to remove or lock away dangerous items and seek some professional help until you find a longer-term solution.
>
> If you are physically safe then the best way to cope with agitation and verbal aggression in the moment is to stay calm and listen to your relative's concerns. Breathe and try not to take the behaviour personally. Try not to respond in a way that might escalate the situation. It's helpful to reassure your relative and show them that you understand their fear, anger or frustration. If the agitation turns into physical aggression, seek assistance or protect yourself by moving to a safe distance from your relative until the behaviour stops.

In the previous chapter, we looked at the fact that cognitive changes experienced by your relative won't always be a direct consequence of the dementia itself. The anxiety and depression that can co-occur with dementia may make it difficult for your relative to think clearly, remember, solve problems and make decisions or judgements. Diminished self-confidence, fear of failure, embarrassment or an unpleasant experience following diagnosis can interfere with an enjoyment of life, making it harder for your relative to do the things they would like to do. These factors may even cause them to withdraw from social situations and activities that would help to preserve their cognitive and day-to-day functioning and add pleasure to their life. Identifying, understanding and treating anxiety and depression can make life less challenging for both of you and make it a lot easier to continue to engage with life and live well with dementia.

These symptoms are most effectively managed when they are precisely described as this will help pinpoint potential triggers. The factors that trigger neuropsychiatric symptoms may be related to you and others involved in your relative's care, to your relative's surrounding environment or to your relative themselves. Identifying the triggers has nothing to do with blame and everything to do with preventing or at the very least minimising the occurrence of neuropsychiatric symptoms. Many of these triggers can be modified or removed, and prevention may be simply a case of removing the offending trigger or may require you and others who interact with your relative to adjust your own behaviour. As care partner, your ongoing observations are critical and the emergence of any symptoms or changing behaviours should be relayed to your relative's medical team, who should use psychotropic treatment (medication) as a last resort and only if non-pharmacological treatments fail. It's important to state here that if symptoms – for example, a hallucination – are not disruptive or unpleasant, and don't bother you or your relative, then that hallucination may not need to be treated.

Learning about neuropsychiatric symptoms will help to increase the likelihood that non-pharmacological treatments will work, preventing the need for pharmacological interventions, which can have serious side effects and negatively impact on your relative's quality of life, their human rights and may also progress their symptoms. Some medications are simply ineffective, while others increase risk of death, or have side effects such as sleepiness, tremor, impaired motor skills and lower blood pressure. Some medications used to treat symptoms such as stiffness and tremors in Parkinson's disease have side effects including hallucinations and psychosis, especially in older patients or those who have had Parkinson's disease for a longer time. Studies suggest that up to 60 per cent of Parkinson's patients might experience some form of mild psychotic symptoms over the course of the disease, with more severe symptoms being less common but still significant. The risk of psychosis often means that adjustments to prescribed medication are required, and this might sometimes include the introduction of antipsychotic medications that do not worsen their Parkinson's symptoms.

You must never stop a medication without consulting the prescribing doctor as suddenly ceasing some medications can have dreadful consequences and can even cause death. Having said that, do enquire why medications are being prescribed, ask about side effects, and discuss non-pharmacological options, other types of medication and any concerns you may have about medicating your relative, particularly when it comes to antipsychotic medications and sedation. Ask for a meeting to discuss how the different drugs your relative has been prescribed may interact, as sometimes doctors can prescribe medications without necessarily taking into account what other medications your relative is on, prescribed by a different doctor.

Before delving into the specifics, I want to share with you some general advice on managing neuropsychiatric symptoms.

Respectful responding

Validation therapy is a compassionate approach that involves empathising with and acknowledging the feelings and experiences of individuals with dementia, rather than challenging or correcting them, to reduce stress and enhance communication. The most important thing is to communicate with your relative with empathy and understanding. Remember, these symptoms are also challenging for your relative to cope with. Aim to make them feel heard and do what you can to help maintain their dignity. Listen carefully to the emotions behind their behaviours. This approach will help you to connect and engage with your relative, establish their needs and address those needs, instead of correcting or confronting their behaviour. Essentially, this technique focuses on respectful responses to the reality that your relative is perceiving at any point in time. This will help your relative to feel respected and listened to, which in turn will reduce anxiety and agitation, improve communication, improve their self-worth and strengthen the bonds between you and your relative. Speak in a calm, loving voice. Use eye contact and gentle touch. Ask about specific details to guide the conversation. Steer discussions towards positive past experiences. Focus on their communication to make them feel heard.

When you listen and observe closely, you may find hints about what they need in what they say or how they act. For example, if they keep pulling at their clothes, they may find the clothes uncomfortable, scratchy or too tight. I was thinking about this the other day as I tried on a few different things till I found something that felt appropriate for what I was planning to do that morning. I knew almost instantly I put something on that I didn't want to wear it. I can't imagine how stressed it would make me feel if I had to wear whatever someone else chose to dress me in and not have the ability to express my discomfort. In addition, I often change clothes during the day to suit what I am doing – I may begin the day in a smart dress for an interview about my work, then change into something less formal for writing; later in the day I may change again, adjusting my clothes according to whether I'm going to garden, kayak, walk, do the shopping or chill out on the sofa. Including your relative in decisions about clothes can prevent this issue; so too can checking in shortly after dressing and on and off throughout the day. If your relative keeps opening and closing drawers, ask if you can help them to find what they are looking for. Think about what that might be and offer suggestions by showing various items. Think over past conversations for clues to things they might be anxious about losing. Look in unusual places, as your relative may have hidden important items like watches or jewellery for fear someone may take them. If they say they want to speak with deceased relatives or friends or go 'home' to a house they no longer live in, there is no reason to confront them with the reality that their relatives are dead or that the 'home' they referred is one they lived in when they were first married. Instead, respond empathetically – ask them what they would say to their relative or what they would do if they were home.

I learned this the hard way when Mum told me she couldn't understand why my dad never came to visit her. I replied almost instantly, saying 'Oh Mum, Dad is dead,' and I will never forget the look of shock on my mum's face and the overwhelming grief and sorrow that followed. She asked me so many questions about when it happened, how it happened and much, much more. It was incredibly distressing for all of us. My dad had died suddenly and even my children, who were in their teens, became distressed, re-experiencing our own grief but also bearing witness to my mum's complete devastation and lack of comprehension about how she didn't know. At this point Mum was living in a care home, but she spent most Saturdays and Sundays at home with us, so I spent the rest of the day using distraction and other means to shift her attention. By late afternoon, our approach seemed to have worked. We were taken by surprise on returning her to the care home around 9 p.m. that evening when she blurted out to the nurses that her Pat (my dad) was dead and the tears flowed again.

That was a huge learning curve for me. It served to remind me that beneath the memory loss (she had forgotten that Dad had died several years before) was a complex individual trying to make sense of the world (why doesn't Pat visit me) who was then capable of not only terrible grief but also had the ability to mask her feelings (she fooled me into thinking that my efforts to distract her had allowed her to return to a place where she had forgotten that Dad was dead). I'd allowed myself to think that Mum's dementia symptoms meant she was – I struggle to find a way to explain this – somehow less complex, simpler, maybe even one-dimensional. I'd forgotten that she had an inner world, an inner voice that tried to make sense of the world, that was also capable of outward behaviour at odds with her inner distress. It's well worth reminding yourself to treat your relative with a dignity that acknowledges them as complex beings. Try to validate their feelings and experiences and do what you can to take practical steps to meet their needs.

Adapting

The human brain naturally resists change, triggering fear responses that lead to fight, flight or freeze reactions. However, it also has a remarkable capacity for resilience and adaptation. Dementia caregiving is a process that requires your adaptation to the ongoing changes to your relative's abilities, behaviours and perceptions of reality. This adaptability is essential for your well-being.

Adapting to change is a fundamental human trait, honed over a lifetime, from early school experiences to major life events like starting a job or becoming a parent. Our ability to adjust, often in subtle ways, allows us to manage daily challenges and significant life events, whether it's modifying plans due to weather or redefining your self after a divorce. This capacity for ongoing adaptation allows us to not only survive unimaginable challenges but to thrive, grow and experience fulfilment. Our ability to adapt to the complexities of life is at the core of human resilience. Adaptability allows us to thrive in the ever-changing world we inhabit.

Despite this adaptability, change remains challenging, especially when unexpected and unwelcome, as in dementia. This can lead to stress and negative emotions. While the brain can adapt, it naturally favours predictability to maintain internal balance, making sudden change unsettling.

Adaptive behaviour allows individuals to effectively adjust to their environment, supporting survival and well-being. Evolutionarily, adaptive behaviours – such as social cooperation and response to threats – enhance our fitness for survival, increasing our ability to thrive in changing environments.

Adaptive behaviour also commonly refers to actions, skills and behaviours that we develop over the course of our lifespan and use in order to perform basic skills and be able to cope with novel situations. Social skills, practical skills and conceptual skills (for example, money, time, numbers) are considered adaptive behaviours. As we learn and develop across our lives, patterns of adaptation emerge. A positive adaptive pattern is where we adjust to a change in a way that results in outcomes we value, such as growth, health, happiness and nourishment. Examples of adaptive behaviours are:

- **Problem-solving**: Facing a challenge by breaking it down into manageable steps and tackling each one systematically. This behaviour helps individuals overcome obstacles in a constructive way.

- **Seeking support**: When feeling stressed or overwhelmed, reaching out to friends, family or professionals for help. This allows people to manage emotions and gain new perspectives.
- **Time management**: Organising daily tasks and responsibilities in a way that balances work, rest and leisure. Effective time management helps individuals achieve their goals and maintain well-being.

These examples highlight how adaptive behaviours contribute to growth and resilience.

Unfortunately, that is not always the case. Maladaptive patterns may emerge that result in short-term gain but ultimately actually hinder us from growing and changing and prevent us from navigating the world in a healthy way. Maladaptive behaviours are a common coping mechanism employed by people of all ages at times of change or distress. Let's take avoidance coping (aka avoidant coping) as an example.

- **Avoidance coping**: This is a way people deal with stress or difficult emotions by avoiding the problem rather than confronting it and dealing with it directly. Instead of facing the issue head-on, a person might try to ignore it, deny it or escape from it in some way. This can provide temporary relief but often makes the problem worse in the long run because it allows the issue to grow, causing greater stress later on.
- **Procrastination**: Delaying tasks until the last minute to avoid discomfort or anxiety related to the task. Though it may relieve immediate stress, procrastination can lead to increased pressure and reduced quality of work over time.
- **Self-isolation**: Withdrawing from social interactions as a way to cope with stress or anxiety. While it might feel safe in the moment, prolonged isolation can lead to loneliness, depression and a decline in social skills.

Understanding avoidant coping and recognising when you're using it can be the first step towards adopting healthier ways to manage the stress and emotions that you encounter on your journey as a care partner. People might use avoidant coping because it feels easier or less painful than addressing the root cause of their stress or anxiety.

Avoidant coping involves strategies that steer clear of dealing directly with stressors or emotional pain. These strategies can include both mental and behavioural avoidance such as procrastination, denial, distraction, substance use, sleeping, self-isolation, overeating or undereating, daydreaming or fantasising.

FATIMA AND KAMAL

Kamal and Fatima have been married for over fifty years. Kamal was diagnosed with dementia a couple of years ago, and Fatima has taken on the role of his full-time care partner. The adjustment has been challenging for both, especially Fatima, who loves her husband dearly but often feels overwhelmed by the responsibilities and emotional strain. Fatima often finds herself feeling anxious and stressed about Kamal's condition. She worries about his frequent confusion and the strain it places on their relationship. When stressed, Fatima tends to adopt avoidant coping strategies.

She procrastinates by putting off scheduling doctor appointments for Kamal, hoping his symptoms might improve on their own. She tells herself that he just needs a bit more rest or a change in routine, even though deep down she knows he needs more professional care. Fatima often denies the severity of Kamal's condition. When friends and family ask how they're managing, she insists that everything is fine, avoiding the reality of their struggles. She finds it easier to pretend things are normal than face the truth. Fatima distracts herself from her concerns and worries by spending hours cleaning the house meticulously during the day and by watching TV while munching on chocolate in the evenings. The satisfaction from cleaning and the enjoyment of TV and chocolate keep her mind off Kamal's deteriorating memory and the decisions she needs to make. These distractions provide temporary relief, but the underlying issues remain unresolved.

While avoidant coping can offer immediate relief, it often leads to greater stress and anxiety over time. Problems that are ignored or avoided don't usually resolve on their own and can become more significant or complicated. Additionally, relying on avoidant coping can prevent people from developing healthier coping mechanisms that involve addressing and managing stress directly. You may recall from section 1 that it's far healthier to adopt coping strategies that involve problem-solving, support, meditation or mindfulness and physical exercise. Check out the ideas on page 103.

FATIMA AND KAMAL

Fatima's eldest daughter, Amira, isn't fooled by Fatima's protestations that everything is fine. One Sunday afternoon, after a family dinner, Amira has a heart to heart with her mum, who eventually agrees that she can't keep on avoiding the reality of the situation. Fatima promises her daughter – and herself – that she will do her best to adopt healthier strategies to manage her stress, which will hopefully boost her own well-being and help her to support Kamal more effectively.

Fatima starts by making a list of all the tasks and challenges she and Kamal face. With the help of Amira, Fatima prioritises them and tackles each issue one by one. For instance, she schedules regular doctor appointments and consults with specialists about Kamal's care plan. Fatima joins a local support group for carers of dementia patients. Sharing her experiences and listening to others in similar situations provides her with emotional support and practical advice. Amira has already agreed to help and so Fatima reaches out to her other adult children, asking for their help with some of the caregiving duties. Fatima begins practising mindfulness meditation for a few minutes each day. She can't manage longer than that but she does find that these moments of calm help her manage her anxiety better and help her to stay present in her daily tasks. She has also learned some

> breathing exercises to use during particularly stressful moments, understanding that Kamal's behaviours are distressing for him too.
>
> Recognising the importance of self-care, Fatima starts going for a 30-minute walk in the morning while a neighbour looks after Kamal. She listens to a book while walking and makes sure that she adopts a brisk pace. These 30 minutes have become very precious to Fatima. She enjoys the break and the 'me time' and finds that it really lifts her mood and reduces her anxiety. She doesn't like to miss a day, but when she does she can really notice the difference. By adopting these healthier coping mechanisms, Fatima finds that she is better equipped to care for Kamal and manage the challenges they face together. Life is not perfect and sometimes she slips back into old habits but overall she feels more in control and less overwhelmed, and their days are filled with more moments of connection and understanding.

Anxiety

Anxiety is a natural, adaptive reaction that we all experience from time to time. It is an alerting signal that focuses our attention and prepares our bodies for action. A healthy amount of anxiety keeps us safe. Healthy feelings of anxiety usually subside when we deal with the stressor or change how we respond to the stressor. For some people, the feelings don't subside. If your relative continuously feels that something awful is going to happen, it becomes very difficult for them to manage their feelings. Ongoing anxiety can interfere with their ability to cope even with small day-to-day challenges. This persistent anxiety makes it harder to think clearly and negatively impacts physical and mental health. Anxiety can stem from not feeling in control, so following a dementia diagnosis it's not surprising for you and your relative to feel anxious. When we don't know what to expect and feel like we can't plan for something or prevent it, that uncertainty can make us anxious.

PERCY AND FLO

Flo was used to her husband's bouts of anxiety. In the early years of their marriage, she'd learned that Percy liked to be alone when he felt stressed or anxious. They'd managed well and in more recent years he became anxious less frequently. Despite this, Flo wasn't surprised when Percy became anxious following his diagnosis. I mean, who wouldn't? She felt overwhelmed and anxious herself. Unlike Percy, who went into himself and shut down, Flo talked her feelings, fears and worries through with her sisters and her friends. This is something she had always done instinctively. Talking things through helped her to feel less alone and often she came away with a different perspective or even a solution. This time was no different; the strong women in her life had really helped her to come to terms with Percy's diagnosis. Of course, she wished things were different, but they helped her to reach a level of acceptance from where she could start to plan for the future rather than wasting energy in futile wishing for the past or mourning what might have been.

Early in their 40-year marriage, Flo learned that it was best not to force Percy to talk and not to take the irritability that inevitably accompanied his anxiety personally. She also learned to tune out his pacing and fidgeting. But since his diagnosis she was struggling with the fact that he had begun to follow her everywhere. It seemed like he was afraid to be alone, which was very different from how he'd dealt with his anxiety in the past. Flo found herself biting her tongue to stop herself from snapping at him for persistently following her and for his never-ending need for reassurance. She felt like she no longer had any personal space; sometimes she felt like she couldn't breathe and was starting to feel a bit frazzled herself. When Percy complained of a racing heart, nausea and diarrhoea, she decided it was best to take him to see their family doctor. At Percy's request, she accompanied him into the surgery. When Percy slipped out to the bathroom to provide a sample, the doctor asked, 'How are things going? How are you both coping?' Her words were weighty, loaded with knowing. True to form, Flo seized the opportunity for

> support; she expressed her concerns about Percy's anxiety and her own inability to cope with his clinginess. The doctor explained to them both that she was pretty sure that Percy's palpitations, nausea, diarrhoea, clinginess, irritability, pacing and fidgeting were all manifestations of his anxiety. Once tests for infection and other possible causes came back negative, she asked Percy and Flo to come back in for a chat. While Percy still possessed sufficient awareness to know that he needed help, he didn't feel comfortable speaking about his anxiety with his doctor, Flo, or indeed anyone he knew. He agreed to give psychological therapy a go. He struggled with talking therapy, but with a supportive family and GP he explored other avenues and eventually discovered that musical therapy with a qualified therapist reduced his anxiety-related symptoms.
>
> The upshot of this was that Flo and Percy came to realise that Percy's anxiety was really interfering with his cognitive abilities. Once his anxiety was better managed, he was able to think more clearly, make decisions and solve problems. He also discovered that the anxiety had been interfering with his ability to concentrate and remember. This realisation, in turn, made him less anxious and better able to make the most of his preserved cognitive functioning.

Being aware of your relative's risk for developing anxiety may help you to address the issue or seek support before it becomes severe or difficult to manage. If your relative has had anxiety in the past, then – like Percy – they are more likely to experience it with dementia. This doesn't mean they *will* experience it, it just means that they are more likely to experience anxiety than someone who has no history of it. Anxiety is also more common in people with dementia who are aware of and have good insight into their condition.

Knowing the type of dementia your relative has matters. Anxiety is particularly common in people with vascular or frontotemporal dementia, less so in people with Alzheimer's disease. People with vascular dementia tend to have more insight into their condition than individuals with Alzheimer's disease, which goes some way towards explaining why anxiety is more common in people with vascular dementia. In the early stages of dementia, both you and your relative may experience anxiety that is directly related to the diagnosis and worry about symptoms, what might be lost and the future. This is a good time to use these feelings of anxiety to spur you to take action to address your concerns proactively.

What you can do

Listening to and acknowledging your relative's worries is a great approach when anxiety is mild. So too is providing realistic reassurance. Anxiety in the first instance is best managed through activity and engagement. Medication may be useful in more persistent or serious cases. Remember that you don't have to deal with this alone. Reducing anxiety often involves the support and skills of a wide range of people. Many people with more severe and persistent anxiety may prefer to speak with a therapist rather than a supportive relative, friend or their GP.

If your relative is experiencing mild to moderate anxiety in the early to middle stages of dementia, there are several ways that you, as care partner, can ease their anxiety. Encourage your relative to engage in physical activity. Staying active not only provides a means to 'work out' stress, it also has the added benefit of improving sleep, which is important since poor sleep can make stress and anxiety worse. Schedule time for a walk every day. Spending time in nature can really help with anxiety. If your relative is willing and you have access to group activities, additional benefits can be gained from engaging in group exercises like dancing.

Neuropsychiatric symptoms

When you say to people that your relative has Alzheimer's disease or any other type of dementia, they will often assume that memory loss or other cognitive symptoms are the most challenging aspects of the disease. However, neuropsychiatric symptoms, which include agitation, aggression, apathy, depression, disinhibition, sleep disturbances and psychosis, are often far more troubling and disruptive. These symptoms make it more difficult for the individual to function on a day-to-day basis and more likely that they will transition to a nursing home. If your relative does things that worry you, says things that are out of character, sees or hears things or has difficulty sleeping, they may well be experiencing neuropsychiatric symptoms. The chances of such symptoms appearing increase as the disease progresses and are more likely to occur or worsen in the late afternoon or evening, a phenomenon known as sundowning (see page 219).

Agitation and aggression

Agitation and aggression are common challenges in dementia care, often stemming from unmet needs, confusion, or changes in the brain, and understanding their triggers is key to providing compassionate support. In addition to the general advice on keeping you and your relative safe on page 199 this section includes suggestions and advice that may help you to manage and minimise the incidence of agitation and aggression.

Keeping a diary can help you to identify any unmet needs, causes or triggers of aggression or agitation. Removing a cause, meeting a need or modifying a trigger could eliminate or at the very least reduce the incidence of a behaviour, making life less challenging for you and your relative. It really is trial and error. Having a written record will help you to identify patterns and narrow down potential triggers. It is critical to look beyond the behaviour itself to identify triggers and contributing factors. These notes will also help you to become familiar with early signs of agitation so that you can act before the behaviour escalates. Keeping a log can also help you identify things that lead to contented, calm and happy behaviours. With time, patience and systematic observation, recording and interpretation of your relative's behaviour through diary-taking will enable you to maximise contentment and happiness and minimise behaviours that are a challenge.

Here are some ideas to consider when you're trying to interpret agitation or aggressive behaviours:

- Could their physical surroundings be too hot or too cold? Could it be too bright or too dark, too noisy or too quiet?

- Are their clothes comfortable? Do they dislike what they are wearing? Do they dislike the feel of the material? Is the waistband or collar too tight?
- What about dentures? Have they become uncomfortable? Gums shrink with age – when was the last time a dentist checked the dentures to ensure they still fit comfortably?
- What about hearing aids? Are they working properly? Are the settings suitable for the environment?
- Can your relative see well? Do they need new glasses? Is the lighting in their room adequate? Do they need their vision or eye health assessed?
- How is their physical health? Could they be experiencing pain or discomfort that they cannot communicate? Your relative's doctor should be able to help by carrying out a medical exam to identify any potential health problems, broken bones or medical causes of discomfort or pain.
- What about their mental health? Could they be anxious, stressed or depressed?
- Could they be constipated, could their underwear be soiled? Are they asking to use the bathroom?
- Has something or someone new become a part of their lives? Has something or someone in their environment or routine been changed recently?
- Does the behaviour only occur when they interact with or spend time with a specific individual or when they are being pushed by others to do something – like being washed, dressed or made to eat or wear something they don't like? Are they being asked to do something they now find frustrating?
- Have they perhaps got cabin fever from being cooped up inside? Are they bored? Do they want time alone or time with others, or time outside?
- Do they feel frustrated because decisions are being made about them without asking them? Do they feel they are not being listened to or can't make themselves understood?
- Are they confused about where they are?

- Are they lonely? Do they miss doing things that they love? Are they being overstimulated by too many visitors and too many activities?
- Conversely, are they under-stimulated – do they spend their days on a sofa with little to entertain, amuse, engage or distract them?
- Have they started a new medication? Could it be a side effect or interaction with other medicines? Check your diary to see if the changes coincide with the introduction of new medication or changes to the dose of existing medications. Speak with the prescribing physician if you suspect this may be a contributing or causal factor.
- Could they have a urinary tract infection – have they been going to the bathroom more frequently?

Not everyone with dementia demonstrates aggressive behaviour. However, as the disease progresses, some individuals may behave in ways that can be described as verbally or physically aggressive. They might swear, shout, scream or make threats. They might throw things, hit, pinch, scratch or pull hair. This kind of behaviour is clearly very distressing for you and for your relative.

Agitation is a state of restlessness, irritation or distress, often shown through behaviours like pacing, fidgeting or verbal outbursts. It can be caused by discomfort, anxiety, confusion or an inability to communicate needs, and is common in people with dementia or other cognitive conditions. If you notice these behaviours, it may mean that your relative is worried or has an unmet need.

Aggression in dementia can stem from a range of causes, some directly related to the disease itself and others due to external factors or co-existing conditions. Research indicates that between 20 per cent and 40 per cent of people with dementia experience aggression due to neurological changes caused by the disease itself – these estimates vary, depending on the type of dementia.

Other non-disease factors account for a significant proportion of aggression cases in dementia. Estimates vary but some studies suggest that addressing these external factors can reduce aggressive behaviours in up to 50 per cent of cases. While brain changes due to dementia play a central role in causing aggression, a significant percentage of aggression in people with dementia is also linked to other factors, which can often be managed with supportive care and environmental adjustments. This means that you might be able to reduce aggressive behaviour by identifying and addressing these external causes. Keeping records will help you to determine whether any of the following may be driving your relative's aggressive behaviours:

- **Physical discomfort:** Pain, hunger, dehydration, fatigue or other unmet physical needs can trigger aggressive behaviours, especially if the person cannot communicate their discomfort. Some studies show that unrecognised pain can lead to a two- to threefold increase in agitation or aggression.
- **Medication effects:** Certain medications or interactions can increase irritability or aggression. For instance, sedatives or antipsychotic medications could make your relative more restless and more agitated rather than making them calmer. A review of studies found that medication side effects account for a significant portion (10–30 per cent) of aggression cases in dementia patients.
- **Environmental triggers:** Overstimulating or confusing environments, loud noises, sudden changes in routine or feeling crowded can be distressing for people with dementia, leading to aggressive responses. Research suggests that environmental factors are often an overlooked cause of aggressive behaviours.
- **Emotional distress and anxiety:** Fear, frustration and confusion are common in dementia, particularly if the person struggles to understand what's happening around them. This emotional distress can trigger aggression. Studies highlight that people who experience frequent disorientation or feel their personal space is threatened are more prone to aggression.
- **Sundowning:** Sundowning is often associated with aggression, and studies suggest that up to 20 per cent of people with dementia

exhibit increased agitation and aggressive behaviour during these hours.
- **Depression, anxiety and psychosis:** Dementia is often accompanied by other mental health issues, such as depression or anxiety, which can amplify feelings of frustration or helplessness, leading to aggression. Research indicates that individuals with both dementia and a mood disorder are at higher risk of displaying aggression.

As the disease progresses, your relative may lose the capacity to communicate effectively and find it increasingly difficult to tell you what they need or how they are feeling. Frequently, agitation or aggression are the only way a person with dementia can communicate what they need. This can be extremely challenging for care partners, especially if, prior to diagnosis, you could finish each other's sentences or instinctively knew what the other was thinking or feeling. It's hard to go from that kind of intimate knowing to a situation where your relative can't tell you what they need, and you can't understand why they are behaving aggressively. It is important for you to remember that your relative's behaviour is not malicious or personal. The most important thing is to accept that communication between you has changed dramatically and do your best to commit to learning this new language – one that will help your relative to communicate and you to interpret their needs and feelings without them recoursing to aggressive behaviours.

Ultimately, it's important to acknowledge that you no longer speak the same language together. Dementia constrains your relative so you are the one who needs to learn the new language so that you can understand what your relative is trying to tell you, what they are feeling or what they might need. It's not easy, it takes dogged detective work, but it can be done. It's like cracking a code – you need to do it systematically but when you break the code, the solution reveals itself and the reward is well worth the effort. You need to be observant, always on the lookout for subtle clues and patterns.

AISHA AND LAYLA

Aisha and her sister Layla had always been close, sharing a bond that allowed them to understand each other without words. When Layla was diagnosed with dementia, Aisha became her primary carer, a role she took on without hesitation. She knew for certain that if the situation was reversed, Layla would do the same for her. Despite willingly taking on the role, Aisha still found Layla's behaviour challenging to deal with.

As Layla's dementia progressed, Aisha noticed that her sister's behaviour became increasingly aggressive. Layla would shout, throw objects, and occasionally even pinch or scratch Aisha. These outbursts were not only distressing but also left Aisha feeling helpless and frustrated. Before the disease took hold, Layla was a loving and gentle soul and Aisha knew that her sister wasn't acting maliciously; but still it was difficult and she really wanted to understand why Layla was behaving this way and whether there was anything she could do about it – not just for herself but for Layla too. She knew Layla found her own outbursts distressing.

Aisha decided to take a systematic approach to identify potential triggers. She began keeping a diary, meticulously noting Layla's behaviour and anything else that seemed significant. The sisters were from a large family, who often came to visit. Aisha observed that Layla's aggression spiked when the house was full of their chatty family. It seemed that the noise was irritating her. Aisha started maintaining a calm and quiet environment, reducing the volume of the television, asking family to speak softly or visit in smaller groups rather than all at the same time.

One day, Aisha noticed that Layla was particularly agitated and kept tugging at her clothes. She realised that Layla's blouse had a tight collar, which might be causing discomfort. Switching to looser, softer clothing seemed to make a difference.

Another time, Layla suddenly became extremely restless and aggressive. Aisha took Layla to the doctor, who discovered that

Layla had a urinary tract infection that was causing her significant discomfort. Treating the infection resulted in a marked improvement in Layla's behaviour.

Aisha also noticed that Layla seemed more content after they spent time in the garden. Realising that Layla might be feeling trapped and restless from being indoors too much, Aisha made a point to ensure Layla had regular outdoor time, which significantly reduced her agitation.

With time, Aisha developed a deeper understanding of Layla's new way of communicating. She learned to interpret subtle cues and patterns in Layla's behaviour that indicated her needs and feelings. This not only reduced aggressive outbursts but also improved the quality of their interactions. Aisha became more attuned to the early signs of Layla's agitation, which included fidgeting or a glazing over of her eyes. When Aisha acted on these signs early, by adjusting something in the physical environment – like temperature, light or noise – or by ensuring Layla's comfort, she often prevented the behaviour from escalating.

When Aisha noticed Layla becoming more withdrawn, she consulted a mental health professional, who diagnosed Layla with depression. With appropriate treatment and support, Layla's mood and behaviour improved.

By systematically observing, recording and interpreting Layla's behaviour, Aisha was able to identify triggers and unmet needs, making life more manageable for both. It was still challenging but with hard work, trial and error and a bucketful of patience, they managed – and Aisha found that the rewards of understanding and connection made the effort worthwhile.

Aisha also kept a consistent daily routine, which helped reduce Layla's confusion and anxiety.

Regularity and routine can keep agitation and anxiety at bay. Keeping things like showering, mealtimes and bedtimes to a regular routine can be reassuring. In an earlier chapter, we looked at the importance of cognitive stimulation, but it is really important to balance that with quiet time. Soothing music can also have a calming effect. Pay attention to how your relative responds to music – look out for subtle changes in their facial expression or movement of their hands or feet. Just because your relative enjoys a certain type of music one day doesn't mean they will enjoy it the next. My mum could enjoy listening to a song one day and the next she could ask me to turn it off because it made her feel sad. Watch out for cues; as the dementia progresses, it may be difficult for your relative to tell you whether they are enjoying or loathing something.

What you can do

We all feel anxious when we lose control, feel out of control or feel that control has been taken from us. Allow your relative to keep as much control in their life as possible. Even simple things like letting them choose what they want to wear or eat can make a big difference to their quality of life and agitation levels. Remember the power of human touch: a gentle touch of reassurance, an appropriate empathetic hug or a hand massage can have a wonderful calming effect. Everyone is different, so make sure you monitor your relative's responses – my mum loved me to apply moisturiser and gently brush her hair but your relative might find these things irritating. It is very individual, you really have to hone your detective skills and become super observant. It helps to avoid overstimulating environments and minimise noise and clutter. If you notice some early signs of agitation, distraction with a pleasant activity or change of location may help.

Sundowning

Sundowning (aka sundown syndrome or late-day confusion), where neuropsychiatric symptoms escalate around late afternoon, evening, sunset or night, is common in people with dementia. Sundowning isn't a disease, it is a collection of symptoms and behaviours that occur at a specific time of day from late afternoon through to night-time. Symptoms include confusion, disorientation, anxiety, agitation, aggression, pacing and resistance to redirection. Sundown syndrome can also include screaming, moaning, yelling, mood swings, suspiciousness, delusional thinking and hallucinations. Some of these symptoms are also expressions of dementia, Parkinson's, delirium or sleep disturbances and so are not specific to sundowning. It is the occurrence or exacerbation of the symptoms in late afternoon, evening and night that set them apart.

Sundowning is a descriptive term rather than a clinical diagnosis. Even though the term has been around since the 1940s, there is currently no consensus around a definition or cause. Some researchers question the existence of sundowning as a distinct phenomenon as opposed to a worsening of existing symptoms as the day progresses, in much the same way that we feel sicker at night when we have a cold, flu or other infection.

It really doesn't matter whether it is a worsening of symptoms or a separate phenomenon: from a care partner's perspective, it is very challenging to deal with these symptoms towards the end of the day when you yourself are feeling tired and more easily irritated. This syndrome or exacerbation of symptoms can often be the deciding factor in whether to move a person with dementia into formal care. Understanding potential causes can help you to identify triggers and minimise symptoms, which will lead to a better quality of life for both of you and allow your relative to remain living at home for longer.

The reasons behind sundowning remain poorly understood but it is most likely that a range of different factors contribute, including insufficient exposure to daylight, poor lighting, increased shadows, fatigue, an infection, internal body clock disturbances, fluctuation in hormone levels over the course of the day, hearing or vision loss, pain, boredom, over- or under-stimulation, depression, anxiety or the side effects of prescribed medication.

What you can do

Observe and take notes to see if a pattern emerges – this may help you to identify what might be causing or triggering the escalation of symptoms. There may be multiple factors at play. Read on for some tips that may help you to address the underlying cause and limit or at least minimise the symptoms and associated distress.

People who experience disrupted sleep and spend most of their time indoors away from natural light are more likely to experience sundowning. Excessive tiredness can increase late-afternoon restlessness, so anything you can do to promote sleep will help. Natural daylight plays a critical role in our health and our ability to sleep well. Daylight isn't just nice to have; it's a basic human need. Exposure to daylight first thing in the morning is critical for setting our internal clocks and helps to regulate the sleep–wake cycle. Plan activities with your relative that involve exposure to natural light throughout the day. A few minutes in the garden, on a balcony or even looking out of an open window first thing in the morning helps to align internal body clocks. Multiple exposures to natural daylight throughout the day will help with sleep at night. Follow the sun around the house – move your relative from room to room so that they can absorb as much daylight through the windows as possible.

Low lighting and increased shadows may aggravate sundowning and late-day confusion. Have a look at the environment your relative is spending time in, brighten up dark corners and adjust lighting levels and direction to avoid shadows. Reflective surfaces (e.g. mirrors, TV screens, windows) can sometimes cause confusion. I know I've sometimes frightened myself catching my own reflection in a window on a dark night. Close blinds or curtains once it starts to get dark outside. If your observations indicate that this is the case, consider covering them with dust sheets or cloths of some kind. Invest in some plug-in night lights to avoid complete darkness, which may trigger agitation or fear.

Limit daytime napping if you can, especially from the late afternoon onwards. Your relative can get some daytime rest if needed but keep naps short (15–20 minutes) and to the early part of the day. While it might be tempting to let your relative take long naps to give yourself a break, it can be counterproductive, leading to disrupted sleep and an increased likelihood of sundowning. To counteract that mid-afternoon sleepiness, schedule a daily outdoor walk, stretches, chair exercises or even a bit of dancing around the time your relative is inclined to nap. Exercise gets the blood flowing and physical activity raises dopamine, noreadrenaline and serotonin levels, which boosts focus and attention.

Check whether your relative might be in pain; could they be hungry, thirsty or uncomfortable? Be conscious of any needs they might have. Try to limit caffeine and sugar consumption to mornings – read the labels, as you'd be surprised how frequently they pop up. Discourage consumption of alcoholic drinks as they can make confusion and anxiety worse. Alcohol may also interfere with medication your relative is taking, increasing side effects or even stopping the medication working. If you are concerned, your GP or pharmacist should be able to advise you about whether it is safe for your relative to drink alcohol.

While on the one hand it is important to keep your relative engaged and active, it is important not to overstimulate or exhaust them. With time, observation and trial and error, you should find a level of activity that provides just the right amount of stimulation to avoid boredom, overstimulation and sundowning. Introducing a regular, predictable routine for waking, meals, walks, daylight exposure and bedtime can bring about feelings of calm.

Creating a calm environment in the evening can sometimes make a difference. Reducing background noise and steering clear of exercise or highly stimulating activities might help. Although watching TV might feel like a natural way to unwind, it can sometimes be unsettling or confusing for people with dementia. Consider gentle alternatives, like playing soft music or soothing sounds. If your relative enjoys it, you might try applying moisturising creams, giving a gentle hand massage, or soaking their feet in warm water to help them relax. If you think pain, an infection, or a side effect from medication might be contributing to sundowning, it could be worth checking in with a health professional.

Apathy and depression

Apathy is common in Alzheimer's disease. Depression also occurs in Alzheimer's disease and while it is less common than apathy, it is better researched. Antidepressants are commonly prescribed for depression in dementia, even though there is little evidence that they are effective and may even be harmful for people with dementia because they are associated with an increased risk of falling, hospitalisation and death. Despite this, over a quarter of people living with dementia in the UK take antidepressants. Apathy and depression can co-occur and can be confused with each other due to some overlapping symptoms, but they are distinct conditions.

Apathy

Apathy is more than laziness or disinterest – it is a medical condition that can be a complication or symptom of Parkinson's disease and stroke as well as Alzheimer's disease. Apathy affects 49 per cent of people with Alzheimer's disease and 72 per cent of people with frontotemporal dementia.

SOPHIE, MARGARET AND JAMES

Sophie sits in the kitchen, watching her mother, Margaret, stare blankly out of the window. Sophie had always admired her mother's seemingly limitless energy. An only child, Sophie was born when Margaret and James were in their mid-forties. Despite being older than all the other mums when Sophie was at school, Margaret was always the most vibrant and energetic. She was always doing something; she always had some project or other on the go and was involved in almost all the local community activities. Sophie's dad used to call her the Energizer Bunny because she just kept on going and going. When Margaret was diagnosed two years ago, she said: 'I'm not going to let dementia stop me from doing the things I love' – and she was true to her word until about three months ago, when she seemed to lose interest in everything. She's gone from high energy to static apathy. Now she mainly just sits there in the blue chair in the kitchen, staring into space. She seems to have no desire to do anything and has lost interest in everything, she has no power, no drive: 'It's like someone has taken my mum away and left a listless empty body.' Sophie feels that 'this is much harder to deal with than the initial diagnosis'.

When Sophie asks her mum if she would like to go for a walk, Margaret doesn't acknowledge the question, she doesn't even glance

> Sophie's way, she just keeps staring out of the window. Sophie's heart sinks every time, and she is finding it increasingly difficult to cope with her mum's non-responsiveness despite Sophie's enthusiastic efforts to get her mum out of that blue chair. Sophie doesn't know what to do and she really misses her mum, who would have jumped at the chance for a stroll in the park.
>
> Sophie's father, James, looks like he has the weight of the world on his shoulders. He had been managing fine, Sophie had been a great help, getting stuck in with the practical stuff. However, since Margaret has become so listless and disinterested, he is struggling to manage her care and his own grief, which seems to have become worse rather than better. He tries to cajole his wife into helping him with their now too large garden – he finds it both hard and sad when she just stares straight ahead, ignoring him. It hurts. It is genuinely painful. It feels like rejection by the person you love most in the world. Both Sophie and James know it's not Margaret's fault, they know she's not made a choice to act this way, but it's still tough.
>
> James feels dreadful when she barely acknowledges his presence. He misses their conversations, her smile, the way she used to light up a room. Every morning, he wakes with optimism, makes her breakfast, and hopes that today might be different. But Margaret takes a few bites, then pushes the plate away, her face devoid of expression. He tries to engage her in activities she once enjoyed, but she seems disinterested in everything. James read up on apathy, he understands intellectually that it isn't Margaret's fault. But emotionally, it is a different story. The woman he loves is physically right next to him, but he can't reach her. He feels guilty for how he feels and for snapping when he is just too exhausted to be patient.

Apathy can be extremely hard to witness because it feels like you are losing the person you love. It's also difficult to support your relative if they seem to have given up, never reward you with a smile or a laugh and no longer care what happens to them or anyone else.

From a professional healthcare perspective, apathy describes a lack of motivation and the absence of goal-oriented action. People with apathy don't express emotions, don't act spontaneously and lack interest in general. We often consider apathy to be the opposite of empathy, but from a medical perspective it's more than that – it's a lack of motivation and interest in general and it's something over which those affected have no control.

If your relative expresses any of the following, they may have apathy:

- **Withdrawal:** Your relative may sit for long periods staring into space. They may stop engaging in hobbies or be less interested in joining conversations or listening to others. They might still enjoy these activities if encouraged or pushed gently.
- **Indifference:** They are no longer concerned about their own condition. Neither are they concerned about no longer participating in activities they once loved. This change is often more noticeable to family members.
- **Dependency:** They might rely on others to suggest and organise activities and to carry out daily tasks not because they can't do them, but because they lack the drive.
- **Emotional blunting:** There's a noticeable reduction in the expression of emotions, both positive and negative. They may have unemotional responses to news or personal events – they may seem to be uninterested or detached.
- **Low energy:** They may also appear to have no energy or motivation to do routine or daily tasks, such as brushing their teeth or having a shower, and may sleep a lot during the day.

Some of these symptoms overlap with those of depression, such as losing interest in things and lacking energy. This is why it can be hard, even for a doctor, to know whether a person has depression or apathy. The main difference between the two conditions is that depression involves more negative feelings, such as sadness or guilt.

RICHIE AND THOMAS

Richie had been caring for his husband, Thomas, since his diagnosis of Parkinson's disease three years ago. Unlike Sophie and John, Richie had found a way to better manage his husband's apathy, though it hadn't been easy. He had joined a support group early on, seeking advice from others who were in similar situations. He'd provided peer support before and volunteered for an LGBTQIA+ support organisation, so it seemed like a natural step for him to seek support for himself as a care partner.

One sunny afternoon, Richie decided to take Thomas to the park. 'Tommy boy, let's go feed the ducks,' he said cheerfully, knowing that Thomas wouldn't show much enthusiasm. Thomas's face was expressionless, but Richie detected a slight, almost imperceptible nod. Richie helped Tommy to dress and got him into the car with little resistance. At the park, Richie held the bag of bread and started feeding the ducks. He handed a piece of bread to Thomas, guiding his hand gently. Thomas followed Richie's lead, his actions mechanical. But Richie noticed a slight change, a softening in his eyes, a faint trace of engagement.

Richie had learned to celebrate these small victories. Instead of focusing on what Thomas no longer did, he cherished the moments of connection they still had. After feeding the ducks, they sat on a bench, and Richie talked about his day. Thomas listened quietly, and though he didn't respond much, Richie knew Thomas appreciated his presence.

Back at home, Richie kept a routine that included activities his husband could still enjoy, like listening to his favourite music or flipping through photo albums. He also made sure to take breaks and care for himself, understanding that his own well-being was crucial in being an effective carer.

Richie's approach wasn't perfect, and there were still many difficult days. But by seeking support and focusing on what they could still share, he found a way to cope with his beloved husband's apathy, maintaining a sense of connection and purpose in their lives.

What you can do

Apathy can be quite tricky to handle. Talking therapies are not really effective, and while doctors might sometimes prescribe antidepressants for someone with apathy, there's not much evidence that these medications help people with Alzheimer's, mixed dementia or vascular dementia. It's generally believed that the best approach is to encourage the person to stay as active as possible and help them keep their confidence up. Creating safe spaces where your relative can try new activities or chat with people without worrying about getting things wrong is crucial. It's also important to ensure that their dementia isn't something they feel ashamed of. Even if they struggle to actively participate in these activities, just being involved can be beneficial. Activities specifically designed for people with dementia can be a great help. Think about joining a local 'Singing for the Brain' group or a dementia café. These are often advertised in local newspapers or community newsletters. Alternatively, contact your local dementia adviser or adult social services to find out what's available in your area. There are various types of structured therapy delivered by trained professionals, such as music therapy, group art therapy, reminiscence therapy, as well as cognitive stimulation therapy discussed in the previous chapter. However, these therapies aren't always available everywhere.

- Music therapy is a therapeutic approach that uses music to address physical, emotional, cognitive and social needs. For people with dementia, listening to or creating music can help reduce agitation, improve mood and evoke memories, making it a powerful tool for connection and relaxation.
- Group art therapy involves creating art in a supportive group setting with a therapist's guidance. This therapy provides a way for people to express themselves creatively, which can be especially helpful for those who struggle with verbal communication. For dementia patients, it can foster social interaction, reduce isolation and promote a sense of achievement.
- Reminiscence therapy encourages people to recall and share memories from their past. This may involve discussing old

photos, familiar objects, music or personal stories. For people with dementia, reminiscing can help stimulate memory, foster social connections and enhance self-worth by focusing on positive experiences and achievements from their life.

Not everyone will like being organised into activities, but it may help to find tasks and activities that your relative enjoys and finds meaningful. Establish a basic daily routine to provide a reassuring structure. Plan a weekly routine with activities that suit your relative's preferences and personality, like group sessions or visiting the park. Identify activities they can contribute to and feel in control of. This helps rebuild lost confidence. Local support groups offer a place where dementia symptoms are understood, and there's no need to worry about embarrassing mistakes. Try to apply these principles at home by staying calm and not getting upset when mistakes happen.

It's helpful to break tasks down into smaller, manageable steps rather than trying to do everything at once. Maintaining simple skills can boost a sense of achievement and improve self-esteem. Try to avoid blaming your relative for being 'lazy', unhelpful or uncaring. Apathy isn't a conscious choice. If you feel frustrated, try to remain calm.

The main thing is to be patient and encouraging. It's tempting to take over, but this can knock your relative's confidence and lead to a loss of important skills over time. Focus on what they achieve, not on what they can't do. Imagine your relative used to enjoy making tea, but now struggles with the steps. Instead of making the tea for them, you could guide them through each step: filling the kettle, switching it on, placing the tea bag in the cup, and so on. Offering gentle prompts and encouragement at each stage allows them to complete the task mostly on their own. Praising them for each step they accomplish reinforces their sense of achievement. By breaking down the task and offering support, you help them maintain their confidence and skills, rather than taking over and unintentionally making them feel dependent or incapable.

Effective communication helps you understand their needs better. Caring for someone with apathy can be very challenging. It's hard to see a loved one seemingly indifferent to what happens to them or those around them. Remember, you're not alone, and there are resources and support systems available to help you through this journey. Seek medical advice: if you notice signs of apathy, it's essential to consult a healthcare provider, who will assess if there are underlying causes of apathy such as depression, pain, sleep disturbances or medication side effects, as these can sometimes be addressed or managed. They may also evaluate whether apathy is related to the progression of dementia itself or if there are co-existing conditions that could be contributing. Certain medications, especially some antidepressants or antipsychotics, can contribute to apathy in some individuals with dementia. The healthcare provider may review current medications to see if adjustments are needed. They might also suggest local support groups or be able to provide you with strategies to manage apathy, such as breaking tasks into small steps, setting up a routine and using gentle encouragement without pressure.

Caring for someone with apathy can be extremely emotionally taxing. Ensure you take time for yourself and seek support when needed. Self-care is key. I'd recommend you join support groups where you can share experiences and gain advice from others in similar situations. Get professional help where you can and don't hesitate to consult a mental health professional if you find the situation overwhelming. Doing this is a sign of strength, not weakness.

Depression

Depression and depressive symptoms often fall under the umbrella of behavioural and psychological symptoms of dementia (BPSD). This is because the brain changes caused by dementia can directly affect how people feel and perceive emotions, leading to depression. Additionally, being diagnosed with dementia brings about significant fears, worries and real losses, which can significantly impact on mood and emotions. Losing cognitive abilities is a big threat to personal identity, especially in the early stages of the disease, but this threat can continue as the disease progresses. If individuals can't handle these stresses, they may develop hopelessness and depression as a reaction.

Some people with dementia are unaware of their worsening symptoms throughout all stages of the disease. This lack of self-awareness can be partly due to brain changes caused by dementia and is known as anosognosia. It is unusual for patients with a dementia diagnosis to have both anosognosia and depression at the same time; it is possible that this lack of awareness protects them from depression. People who are very aware of their cognitive decline, especially right after diagnosis, need a lot of understanding and emotional support from their family and friends. Your support may help them cope better with the diagnosis and illness, which can prevent depression from developing.

The symptoms of major depression in a person with dementia are pretty much the same as the symptoms experienced by people without dementia. In addition to low mood, the person might be irritable, angry or anxious. Changes to sleep, appetite and energy are common and the person may become negative or believe that life has no meaning, purpose or value. If they develop this nihilistic view, they might feel that nothing really matters or that there's no point to things like morality, goals or relationships. In other words, nothing matters.

In addition to feelings of hopelessness, worthlessness and guilt, they may try to self-harm. Cognitive symptoms of depression are difficult to distinguish from symptoms of dementia because some signs of major depression overlap with those of dementia. A major depressive episode generally develops over weeks or months and is a significant new impairment, while dementia develops slowly over months or years. Depression can also make cognitive issues and behavioural changes worse.

If your relative has a history of depression they will be more likely to experience it again, especially if they've had multiple bouts in their lifetime. Becoming aware of causes, risk factors and symptoms can help you figure out what could be contributing to your relative's depression and how to manage it. These might be past traumas, upsetting events, health issues (cardiac issues, chronic pain, hormonal imbalance), or the side effects of medication (sleeping tablets, steroids, medication prescribed for Parkinson's). A lack of meaningful activities or social support, poor sleep quality and excessive alcohol consumption can also make your relative – and indeed yourself – more vulnerable to depression. Older adults might show different symptoms, such as agitation or health anxiety, and physical symptoms such as aches and pains, which depression can worsen.

What you can do

If depression is suspected, it's important to take it seriously. Alarming as it sounds, it is important to be aware that dementia can increase suicide risk, particularly soon after diagnosis. If you're concerned about your relative, reach out to your GP, a member of your relative's healthcare team, the Samaritans or other support services. Treatments vary, based on the severity and duration of depression. For mild cases, you can encourage your relative to connect with support groups or your GP might recommend self-help strategies your relative could adopt with your support. More severe cases could involve antidepressant medications and talking therapies. Despite the challenges dementia poses, talking therapies can be beneficial, especially in the early stages. Support groups can also offer solace by connecting people with similar experiences.

There are basic rights and freedoms, commonly called 'human rights', that each and every one of us have, simply because we are human. These are things that everyone deserves, like the right to be safe, treated fairly, respected, and allowed to make our own choices. Human rights protect us from being treated badly and help ensure everyone is treated with dignity and respect, no matter who they are. Your relative and others with dementia are at risk of having their basic rights overlooked or denied because the disease can affect their ability to communicate and advocate for themselves.

For this reason, it is critical that you and anyone else who interacts with or cares for your relative respects their human rights. It is important to be aware of this.

- Involve your relative in decisions and encourage open discussions about their feelings.
- Be patient and understanding if you can; sometimes your relative needs a listener more than advice.

- Encourage, support and facilitate social interaction, whether through group activities or one-on-one time.
- Encourage physical activity, which can help with depression and sleep issues.
- Engage in enjoyable activities, such as reminiscence therapy or creative hobbies.
- Encourage healthy eating and ensure that alcohol and caffeine, if consumed, are consumed in moderation.
- Ensure they stick to prescribed treatments, including medication and therapy.
- Create positive routines and involve your relative in daily tasks to boost their confidence.
- Reduce stress in the environment by making the home more comfortable and less cluttered. A cluttered environment puts extra stress on the brain, making it difficult to focus attention or stay focused amid distractions. This is something worth noting for yourself if you are female, as research suggests that women are more affected by clutter-induced stress than men. It's worth noting that taking tidiness and cleanliness to the other extreme is linked to anxiety. Not all clutter is bad – occasionally it can spark creativity.
- Be mindful of your relative's energy levels; start activities slowly and build up as they're able.

Living with both dementia and depression is tough, but with understanding, support and the right approach, you can make a significant positive impact. Remember, there are dementia supports and advisers ready to provide the help and guidance you need.

Psychosis

Psychosis is characterised by a loss of contact with reality. It is a symptom that can occur in a variety of conditions, including dementia. Psychosis is often associated with hallucinations (seeing or hearing things that are not there) and delusions (holding false beliefs). If your relative is affected, their thoughts, perceptions, behaviours and overall functioning could be significantly impacted. Psychosis and the phenomena associated with it are generally persistent, severe, difficult to manage and unlikely to disappear spontaneously. The use of antipsychotic medications to treat dementia-related psychosis is controversial with regard to safety and their effectiveness to the extent that some countries have restricted, controlled and regulated their use. The good news is that prevention is achievable through accurate diagnosis and careful observation and modification or removal of triggers.

> ### MENTAL OR BEHAVIOURAL CHANGES
>
> The various terms used to describe and categorise different mental or behavioural changes that you may encounter can be very confusing.
>
> **Delusions**
> A delusion is a false belief that a person firmly holds, even when there is clear evidence that it isn't true. For example, your relative might believe that someone is trying to harm them, even though there's no actual threat. If your relative experiences delusions, this dementia symptom can cause them to misinterpret reality in specific ways.
>
> Key point: Delusions are false beliefs that are strongly held despite evidence to the contrary.
>
> **Hallucinations**
> A hallucination is when someone perceives something that isn't actually present. Hallucinations involve the senses, so they can be visual (seeing things), auditory (hearing sounds), tactile (feeling sensations that aren't real), and so on. They are not based on real events or objects.
>
> Key point: Hallucinations are false sensory experiences of seeing, hearing or feeling things that aren't there.
>
> **Delirium**
> Delirium is a sudden and severe change in mental function, marked by confusion, disorientation and difficulty focusing. It often comes

on quickly and may fluctuate throughout the day. Delirium is usually caused by a medical issue, such as an infection, dehydration or reaction to medication, and is usually temporary if treated.

Key point: Delirium is sudden confusion or disorientation, often caused by a medical condition (such as a UTI) and is typically temporary.

Agitation
Agitation is a state of restlessness, irritability or distress that can make a person feel unsettled or lead them to pace, fidget or become verbally or physically aggressive. Agitation can be triggered by factors such as pain, discomfort, unfamiliar environments or difficulty communicating needs. Agitation isn't based on false beliefs or sensory experiences, but rather reflects a general state of discomfort or anxiety.

Key point: Agitation is restlessness or distress, often shown through fidgeting, pacing or irritability, commonly triggered by discomfort or stress.

Hallucinations

Hallucinations involve experiencing things that aren't really there and can affect any of the senses. Visual hallucinations, where people see things that don't exist, are the most common in dementia. These can range from simple visual phenomena like flashing lights to complex scenes involving animals, people or unusual situations.

It's important to note that sometimes individuals with dementia might simply be mistaken about what they've seen rather than be experiencing true hallucinations.

Although hallucinations are one of the most common psychiatric symptoms of Alzheimer's disease, very little research has been carried out to increase our understanding of the complex underlying mechanisms. It is very difficult to pinpoint any single factor as a main contributor to hallucinations in Alzheimer's disease. Alzheimer's disease is a complex condition that involves various cognitive, psychiatric and neurological symptoms. These symptoms can vary widely among individuals, partly due to differences in the presence of plaques and neurofibrillary tangles in different areas of the brain. One theoretical model suggests that hallucinations in Alzheimer's disease are primarily seen in patients with certain underlying traits (e.g. a genetic predisposition, impairment of hearing and sight, cognitive deficits, neurological deficits). These traits, combined with other state-like factors (e.g. side effects of medication, psychological distress) can trigger hallucinations. On this view, hallucinations are not caused by a single factor, such as psychological distress, medication side effects, memory problems, neurological issues or sensory deficits. Instead, they result from the interaction of these various factors. Hallucinations can also be a rare side effect of many medications, including drugs used to treat Parkinson's disease.

To complicate matters further, hallucinations can be caused by physical illnesses like fever, seizures, strokes, migraines and infections. These conditions can interfere with brain function and lead to delirium – a medical emergency, often accompanied by hallucinations. Delirium is discussed later in this chapter.

Visual hallucinations, especially in dementia with Lewy bodies, are often vivid, complex and realistic, involving people or animals, and can last for several minutes. Auditory hallucinations involve hearing sounds, such as voices or footsteps, that aren't there. Although less common, hallucinations can involve the other senses: smelling scents, such as smoke or perfume, that aren't present; feeling sensations, like being touched or insects crawling on the skin, that aren't real; or tasting things that aren't there, such as a metallic taste.

Hallucinations can be distressing and frightening, leading to the need for support. However, some people may find certain hallucinations comforting, depending on their nature and the response of those around them.

Sometimes, what appears to be a hallucination might be a misperception. To differentiate between a misperception and a hallucination, it is important to listen carefully. Try to understand what your relative is describing and check for possible causes. For example, a busy carpet pattern might be mistaken for a swarm of insects.

Ensure hearing aids are functioning properly and schedule hearing checks if auditory hallucinations are suspected. Ensure regular dental visits to rule out issues like tooth decay or denture problems if they report unusual tastes.

If hallucinations occur regularly, arrange a GP appointment. Regular medication reviews are essential as new medications or their combinations can trigger hallucinations.

What you can do

How you respond can significantly affect your relative's experience. Describe what is happening and repeat it calmly if necessary. Avoid arguing. Stay with your relative and reassure them. Ask them to describe their hallucination. Moving to a different location might help if hallucinations are specific to one place. Check your relative's needs. Ensure they are not hungry, thirsty or uncomfortable, as these can contribute to delirium and hallucinations. Employ gentle distraction by engaging them in another activity to see if the hallucination stops. Regular social interaction can reduce the likelihood of auditory hallucinations. Supporting someone with dementia involves understanding and adapting to their reality, offering empathy and appropriate care to ensure their well-being.

If hallucinations involve multiple senses or are frightening, last long or happen frequently, seek medical attention. Whether that is an appointment with your GP or attendance at an emergency department, bring details about:

- What your relative experienced and when it happened.
- The duration and setting of the hallucination.
- How your relative responded and their descriptions.
- Current medications and dosages, including over-the-counter drugs.
- Relevant medical history and use of alcohol or recreational drugs.

Delusions

Delusions are strongly held false beliefs commonly experienced by individuals with dementia. These delusions can manifest as paranoia, causing the person to feel threatened without a valid reason. Dementia often leads to increased suspicion of those around them. Those affected may feel they are being watched or that someone is plotting against them, often jumping to conclusions with little evidence. Dementia impairs their ability to moderate these extreme thoughts and emotions.

> **EMMA AND JUNE**
>
> When Emma pops in to visit her 85-year-old grandmother June, she is surprised to find her usually calm and loving Nana distressed. Before Emma can ask her what is wrong, June launches a verbal attack on Emma, accusing her of taking money from her purse. Despite Emma's repeated protestations, June remains convinced that Emma is the thief. Even after Emma locates June's bag, complete with purse and cash, behind her bathroom door, June is not for turning – she sticks to her guns and says she knows for sure that Emma stole cash from her purse.

Caring for a relative with delusions can be challenging, especially when they are convinced you've done something wrong. It's helpful to remember that their delusions feel as real to them as your reality feels to you. Typically, it's not possible to convince them they are mistaken. If delusions appear suddenly, seek urgent medical advice to rule out delirium. It is important to let your relative's medical team know about the emergence of this new symptom, especially if the delusions are distressing.

> **PIOTR AND AGNIESZKA**
>
> When Piotr moved into his house 25 years ago, he found his neighbour Matthew's constant questions intimidating. With time, he learned that Matthew was just trying to make Piotr feel welcome by showing a friendly interest. But Piotr, who was diagnosed with dementia with Lewy bodies a year ago, has begun to feel that Matthew and his other

> neighbours are plotting against him. He believes they are constantly watching him and waiting for a chance to harm him, even though there is no evidence to support this. Piotr peeks through the curtains, his heart racing. 'They're out there again,' he mutters to himself. His wife, Agnieszka, tries to calm him. 'Piotr, no one is watching us. It's just Matthew tending to his garden.' But Piotr can't shake the feeling of being observed. 'They're planning something, Agnieszka. I can feel it,' he insists, the paranoia gnawing at his sense of safety.

Delusions in dementia arise when a person struggles to piece together information and memories accurately, leading to false beliefs. The likelihood of delusions increases as dementia progresses. Delusions are more prevalent in dementia with Lewy bodies and can also affect individuals with Alzheimer's disease and vascular dementia, particularly in later stages. They are less common in frontotemporal dementia. Delusions in dementia typically fall into two categories: persecutory delusions and misidentifications. Piotr's belief that his neighbours intend to do him some harm is the result of persecutory delusions. If your relative thinks that you are an imposter or someone else or doesn't recognise their home, or themselves in a mirror, their delusions are misidentifications of people or places.

ELEANOR AND TERRY

> Eleanor often mistakes her son Terry for her late husband, Andrew. While this was upsetting for Terry at first, he's grown used to it. Lately, he has noticed that Eleanor seems confused in her sitting room. She keeps asking Andrew (Terry) where her china cabinet is and accuses him of painting the walls without consulting her – she says she much preferred the gold flock wallpaper. When Terry told Eleanor's sister Eve what his mum was saying about the sitting room, Eve recalled that when Eleanor was first married, their china cabinet, a family heirloom, took pride of place in their front room, which Eleanor and Andrew had decorated in gold flock wallpaper.

The most common delusions include:

- **Theft:** Misplacing items and believing they've been stolen. This can also lead them to hide items, which exacerbates the issue.
- **Harm:** Believing those close to them intend to harm them in some way, which can range from putting poison in their food to spouses being unfaithful.
- **Home:** Not recognising their current home, especially if they think it's somewhere they never lived. This can be due to 'time-shifting' (see below), where they recall a past home.

What you can do

Recognise that delusions feel very real to the person experiencing them. It's natural to feel upset and want to correct them, but this often causes more distress. Instead, consider these strategies:

- **Discuss their thoughts:** encourage them to talk about their delusions, which can reveal underlying issues.
- **Acknowledge their feelings:** validating their emotions can prevent escalation and maintain trust.
- **Offer alternative explanations:** gently suggest other possible explanations for their concerns.
- **Reassure them:** ensure they know their concerns are taken seriously.
- **Manage distress:** if a delusion causes significant problems, find ways to minimise distress. For example, if they believe food is poisoned, consider meal delivery options they can trust. If feasible, have them prepare the meals with you or taste the food for them or eat with them.

When a person with dementia makes accusations:

- **Stay calm:** try not to take accusations personally.
- **Consider past confusions:** their accusations may be based on past events.

- **Avoid arguments:** arguing can intensify their distress. Acknowledge their feelings instead.
- **Investigate:** if possible, verify the truth behind accusations without dismissing their concerns.

To reduce the risk of delusions:

- Decide on designated places to keep frequently mislaid items, such as keys, in set places.
- Ensure your relative has up-to-date eye and hearing tests to minimise misinterpretations.
- Maintain familiarity and avoid unnecessary changes in their environment.
- Ensure that their medications are regularly reviewed by your GP, the prescribing professional or other healthcare provider.
- Encourage social engagement and stimulating activities to reduce loneliness and isolation.

Research shows that these strategies can help manage and reduce the impact of delusions in individuals with dementia.

Delirium

If you notice a sudden change in your relative's mental state or behaviour, it is important to consider delirium, which is often the first sign that a person is becoming medically unwell. Delirium is not dementia, although they can appear similar. Delirium is a serious complication of a medical illness that requires medical attention. Older people with dementia are at increased risk of delirium. Unfortunately, delirium can accelerate dementia symptoms. It is, therefore, important to be aware of the signs of delirium so that you can intervene and get medical attention quickly; doing so can prevent deterioration of dementia symptoms. Delirium can manifest in different ways in different people. A person with delirium may:

- Be disorientated.
- Have hallucinations.

- Have delusions.
- Have sudden mood swings.
- Have sudden changes in behaviour,
- Be less alert.
- Be easily distracted.
- Struggle to follow a conversation.
- Speak less clearly.
- Suddenly become unable to do something – like walking or eating.

There are two types of delirium. A person with hyperactive delirium can become overactive, seem restless or agitated, be unable to sit still, respond aggressively or resist care, not know where they are, become wary of other people or have delusions or hallucinations. It is easy to confuse these symptoms with agitation. In contrast, when a person has hypoactive delirium, it may be confused with depression because they may become withdrawn, tired, sluggish, sleepy, struggle to maintain focus when awake, interact less with people and move little. This type of delirium is common in people with dementia; so too is mixed delirium, where people switch from hyperactive to hypoactive throughout the day or from one day to the next.

What you can do

Delirium is characterised by sudden onset and an acute change in mental state, together with fluctuations in awareness or consciousness. As their care partner, you will know when your relative is 'not themself'. Delirium affects a person's ability to sustain attention. A simple test you can do if you are concerned that your relative has delirium is to ask them to squeeze your hand every time you say the letter 'A', then spell out H-A-V-E-A-H-E-A-R-T. If your relative can't follow or misses the 'A', it is a good indicator that they may have delirium, and you should seek immediate medical attention. If you can't get your relative to a doctor, try to get a urine sample from them and ask your GP to test it for infection. Research indicates that UTIs are one of the leading triggers of delirium in older people and people with dementia, primarily because infections can lead to systemic inflammation and affect brain function. Research in nursing homes has shown that residents with dementia who develop delirium often have UTIs as the underlying cause, with some estimates indicating that UTIs contribute to delirium in about 25–30 per cent of cases in these settings. Keep an eye out for common signs of a UTI in your relative (see box below). The earlier delirium is treated, the sooner it should resolve.

> **UTI SYMPTOMS**
> - A need to pee more often than usual.
> - Pain or discomfort when peeing.
> - Sudden urges to pee.
> - Feeling unable to empty your bladder fully.
> - Pain low down in the tummy.
> - Urine that's cloudy, foul-smelling or contains blood.
> - Feeling generally unwell, achy and tired.

Time-shifting

Time-shifting is a phenomenon where a person with dementia seems to experience a different reality. Their perception, though different from yours, is very real to them.

For example, they might not understand recent technology, or might expect friends and family to appear much younger or believe that deceased friends and relatives are still alive. They may also not recognise their own reflection in a mirror because they expect to see a much younger version of themselves.

Memory plays a crucial role in understanding the world around us. The brain combines sensory information with memories to make sense of the present. However, dementia often damages or prevents access to more recent memories, causing individuals to rely more on older memories. For instance, a person with dementia might place an electric kettle on the stove because they remember using a stovetop kettle in the past. Their brain uses older memories to fill in gaps, making them feel as though they are living in the past. Therefore, they may fail to recognise their adult children or other family members, they may struggle with newer technology or misinterpret their surroundings.

Time-shifting is common in Alzheimer's disease and can occur in all types of dementia, becoming more frequent as the condition progresses. Individuals may shift between being time-shifted and present within the same day. If your relative is experiencing time-shifting, they may say they have to pick up the children from school or ask to speak to their mother, recalling early life memories.

What you can do

Correcting a time-shifted person can be distressing. Time-shifting is due to brain damage and is not a choice. Consider these tips to support them:

- **Announce yourself:** saying your name when you enter a room may help to prevent confusion.
- **Listen attentively:** try to understand their reality by paying close attention to their words and actions. Acknowledge their concerns and offer help.
- **Avoid contradicting them:** don't confront their beliefs, as this may cause distress and trigger other symptoms. Choose gentle distraction, which can be effective.
- **Stay positive:** maintain a calm and friendly demeanour, as emotional memories are easier for them to retrieve.
- **Remain calm:** if you feel frustrated, take a break to regain composure.
- **Focus on well-being rather than reality:** your relative with dementia doesn't need to fully understand your reality to feel happy. Join their present and continue with actions that make them content.

These strategies may help to prevent or reduce time-shifting:

- Remove or cover mirrors and shiny surfaces to prevent distress from not recognising their reflection.
- Avoid introducing new technology unless necessary, as they may find it confusing.
- Use familiar items from their past, such as an old-fashioned radio, to reduce confusion.

Supporting a person with dementia involves adapting to their perceived reality with empathy and patience, helping them feel safe and content despite the challenges posed by time-shifting. It is important to note that experiencing one or more of these symptoms does not necessarily mean a person has psychosis. A comprehensive evaluation by a healthcare professional is necessary to determine the underlying cause and appropriate treatment.

The suggestions in this chapter aim to help you to manage your relative's symptoms, improve their overall well-being, and create a supportive and calming environment for your relative if they experience dementia-related psychosis. Since each person's needs and symptoms are unique, a personalised approach can be especially helpful to ensure the best possible outcomes.

CHAPTER 11

Maximising the good stuff

NATALIE

Natalie was a stay-at-home mum. She considered herself lucky to have that option financially. Her husband, Steve, had a very well-paid job and as an only child she was the sole beneficiary of her parents' estate, which was not insubstantial. She loved homemaking and enjoyed every minute of raising her three children. She led an active life, playing tennis a few times a week and walking on the beach with friends almost daily. She was a regular volunteer in community activities and kept her brain ticking over by doing night and online courses in whatever took her fancy.

Of course, like any family they had their moments, but overall they were a happy family that got on well and loved spending time together. When Steve died suddenly in his late forties, the family became even closer, united in their grief and shock. They pulled together and made a concerted, conscious effort to support their mum.

In her early sixties, Natalie noticed some forgetfulness creeping in. More aware of her own mortality following Steve's death and conscious of a family history of Alzheimer's, she began to think about the possibility that she might develop dementia at some point in the future. Always a practical woman, she wanted to be prepared and to face the possibility head-on.

She didn't catastrophise but she didn't like the idea that there might come a time where she wasn't able to indicate her wishes or be involved in important decisions that affected her directly. She shared her concerns over a family Sunday lunch with her adult children. Their initial reactions were of the variety of 'wish my memory was as sharp as yours', 'don't be worrying about something that might never happen' or 'let's cross that bridge if we come to it'. She acknowledged that any issues she had were minor and might amount to nothing but was very firm in articulating her desire to have a say in her own future.

Ideally, she would have preferred not to involve her adult children at that juncture, but she had done a little research herself and discovered that there was no legal way for her to document her wishes (this has subsequently changed). She decided to consult her children about the best way she could make her wishes known. They came up with a plan. They bought a pretty journal for Natalie to record her wishes. At first, she detailed the big things like care, medication, resuscitation and so on. She kept the journal close by and continued to record her wishes over the next few months. Then she put it somewhere safe and told her children, her closest friend and her sister its location, together with an instruction that should dementia or any other condition render her vulnerable or unable to speak on her own behalf, the journal should be consulted.

Natalie continued to engage with and enjoy life for several years before her premonition of dementia was confirmed and before more debilitating symptoms started to emerge. In the later stages of Natalie's dementia journey, whenever there was a decision to be made, instead of discussions and disagreements her adult children simply consulted the journal. This allowed the siblings to present a united front and articulate their mum's wishes with confidence and conviction, safe in the knowledge that this is what their beloved mum, Natalie, truly wanted.

There is no denying that dementia is a devastating disease, but it is genuinely possible to live well with dementia. Acceptance and action are key. Shifting focus from the disease will help you to continue enjoying life despite dementia. Optimising both your own and your relative's physical, mental and brain health is a great way to improve quality of life for both of you, slow the progression of your relative's symptoms and reduce your own risk of developing dementia. In this chapter, there is detailed guidance on how to create a home that supports rather than hinders a person with dementia and an introduction to supportive technologies and other interventions that can help you both to live well despite dementia.

Live well with dementia

Living well with dementia involves a combination of self-care, practical planning, maintaining health and creating a supportive environment with a focus on your relative and on positive experiences. By taking proactive steps and seeking the right support, individuals with dementia and their care partners can lead fulfilling lives.

It's important to prioritise self-care and accept your feelings. It's normal to feel a range of emotions, including shock, sadness, guilt, grief and more. Following the advice in section 1 will help you to manage these feelings and then move on without losing yourself or becoming crushed by the burden of care. Being kind to yourself and seeking support are critical elements of self-care that will help you to live well. Caregiving can improve your health, giving your life greater meaning and purpose. Care partners who can accept the diagnosis, adopt adaptive coping strategies, express gratitude, give and receive support and set boundaries can enjoy health benefits and experience caregiving in a positive way.

After the shock of diagnosis, it is important to accept that dementia is part of your life. Acceptance allows you to focus on the now, to live in the moment. It's also helpful to understand dementia. This is why section 2 provides detailed information about dementia so that you can focus on the person in the present moment, treating them with dignity and respect. With this knowledge, you can empower and support your relative and take action to make life as good as it can possibly be. And it *can* be good – there can be laughter, joy, fun, love, meaning and purpose, all of which bring about happiness and contribute to a life well lived.

Live well now and in the future

Take time with your relative to discuss and document their care preferences, including daily care routines, medical treatment, formal care, etc. This won't be easy and will likely bring up all sorts of emotions and grief, but it is important to do this sooner rather than later while your relative still has the necessary faculties. Having clearly articulated preferences and wishes will reduce stress for everyone involved and will limit family arguments and emotional upheaval. Consult with a legal adviser who specialises in this area to ensure that legal documents (for example, wills, enduring or lasting power of attorney, advance directives) are in place. There is nothing stopping your relative recording less formal everyday preferences, as Natalie did – for example, for food, clothing, activities, music and the use of supportive technology or location devices.

The sections that follow offer suggestions regarding adaptations and tools that may help your relative to better navigate their home and hold on to their independence and functioning for as long as possible. It might be useful to explore these adaptations and tools as early as possible and discuss with your relative with a view to recording their preferences in advance. Remember, 'nothing about you without you'. Involve your relative in decisions that affect them.

Live well at home

Often, loss of function and loss of independence come down to the fact that the person with dementia has difficulty feeling safe and comfortable in their own home. This can happen for several reasons, including memory issues, poor vision, hearing loss, recognition issues, mobility issues or indeed health issues other than dementia.

You can support your relative to maintain independence by adapting their home or your home, if they come to live with you, to take account of these issues and other changing needs. Small changes can make a big difference. You don't need to completely revamp your home following diagnosis; you can gradually make alterations as needs arise or as symptoms dictate.

Dementia can make it difficult for a person affected to recognise where they are or what time of day it is. They may not remember where the bathroom is or what is behind each cupboard in the kitchen. In addition to the perceptual issues that can accompany dementia (e.g. misidentification, hallucinations), older people experience many changes in their vision (e.g. cataracts, macular degeneration) that can add to confusion and influence their ability to navigate their environment safely. With age comes a reduction in the ability to perceive contrast, diminished colour vibrancy (e.g. red might look like a pink) and a loss of the ability to discriminate between various blues or between blue and black. Visual issues can make it difficult for a person with dementia to distinguish between the floor and a step, or a floor and a wall. The fashionable trend to furnish a room in neutral tones that blend seamlessly with the neutral wall coverings is a nightmare for people with dementia because everything just blends, making it impossible for them to navigate – sofas blend into floors and doors blend into walls. Similarly, mood lighting that created a romantic ambience in the past can now cast shadows and create dark corners that induce fear and anxiety and may even trigger behaviours that challenge.

What you can do

- Manipulating light will help orient your relative to time and prevent confusion.
- During the day, keep curtains open and blinds pulled up to give your relative access to as much daylight as possible through the clean windows.
- Remove any items of furniture, ornaments or plants that may block light from entering the room.
- Keep all rooms flooded with daylight throughout the day to help your relative keep track of time.

- Dimmable light fittings are a great way to match your internal artificial light to the natural light cycles, which will help entrain your relative's internal body clock and improve their sleep.
- You may need to invest in some additional lighting to brighten dark corners and avoid shadows that can trigger neuropsychiatric symptoms.
- Avoid stark, bright, institution-style overhead lighting – keep the lighting design pleasant, with a safe, homely feel.
- Close curtains as soon as it gets dark to avoid reflections that may cause distress.
- Complete darkness is best for restorative sleep, but you will also need to ensure a safe passage to the bathroom at night.
- Night lights are great but if, like me, you or your relative find their constant glow disrupts sleep then invest in night lights with sensors set to come on with movement.
- Getting outside in daylight is critical for resetting circadian rhythms so make sure the garden is safe and free from trip hazards.
- Placing family photos around the house will not only act as a memory aid but will also help ground your relative in time. As the disease progresses, you might add labels with people's names.
- Keep regularly used and frequently mislaid items like mobile phones, remote controls, glasses, keys, wallets etc. in a consistent, highly visible place. Perhaps use a tray on a side table next to your relative's favourite chair for remotes, glasses and mobile and a hook in the hallway next to the front door for keys.

Use colour contrast to define your home environment. This will help your relative distinguish between vertical surfaces (e.g. walls) and horizontal surfaces (e.g. floors), making it easier for them to understand and navigate the rooms in their home.

- A cheap and simple way to use colour contrast to distinguish the floor from steps is to stick tape on the horizontal edge of the step that is a different colour from the riser, to mark the transition between levels.

- Paint skirting boards in a colour that contrasts with the wall and the floor.
- Paint the walls in a colour that contrasts with the sofa.
- Choose bedclothes that contrast with the colour of the floor.
- Use plates and cups that contrast with the colour of the tablecloth/top.
- Install light switches and plug sockets that contrast with the walls.
- If the wall covering is dark, use white light switches and sockets.
- If the wall covering is light, use darker switches and sockets.
- If your budget extends to it, consider asking an electrician to move plug sockets to locations that are easier to see and reach.
- Avoid stripes and strong patterns as they cause confusion.
- Solid colours are least confusing for upholstery and soft furnishings.
- If you can't afford to reupholster furniture, a carefully placed plain throw can solve the problem.
- Paintings, wall hangings and mirrors can become problematic as the disease progresses. Monitor your relative's reactions and remove them or hang a dust cloth over them.

A house that was once easy to navigate may become a health and safety hazard due to confusion and changes in perception. Observe your relative as they move about the house – have there been any near collisions with furniture, have there been any trips or falls? Take a close look at the layout, lighting, textures and patterns in each room. A shiny floor that was once your relative's pride and joy might appear slippery and wet, a dark rug might seem like a hole in the ground and some patterns may look like litter. When contrasting colours are used in different rooms throughout the house, a person with dementia may see shadows or misperceive the change in colour as a change in floor level.

- Use the same or similar floor covering in rooms that lead into each other to give your relative the sense that they are walking on a continuous level surface. Plain matt flooring is best.

- Remove floor mats and rugs as they can confuse and cause trips and falls.
- Leave internal doors open between the most used rooms. It will make it easier for your relative to navigate their home.
- Tape down any loose edges on the main floor covering.
- Make sure your relative has a clear pathway in each room so that they can move about freely without risk of falling.
- Remove or adjust the position of any potential trip hazards such as side tables, lamps or coffee tables. However, don't be tempted to change the arrangement of furniture too much. The dementia brain can navigate the familiar better than the new, so just remove or reposition potential hazards.
- Remove clutter as it can overwhelm the dementia brain.
- Seats with arms that are at a suitable height above the ground are the easiest to rise from.
- Painting doors a different colour to their frames will make it easier for your relative to use them. Instead of painting, you can stick coloured tape around the frame.
- Painting the frame and the door the same colour as the wall will make it recede into the wall, making it very difficult for your relative to distinguish one from the other.

Bathrooms can be perceptually confusing and potentially dangerous.

- Install a toilet lid and seat that contrasts with the rest of the toilet.
- Remove clutter.
- Keep everyday items like toothpaste, soap, shampoo and shower gel where they can be seen and reached easily and safely.
- Contrast towels with bathroom walls.
- White sinks can be difficult to see, especially in a bathroom with white tiles. Adding colourful waterproof stickers is a cheap and cheerful way to make the sink easier to see.
- Leave the door to the bathroom ajar when not in use – that way, it will be obvious to your relative where the bathroom is.

- As the disease progresses, you may need to put signs on the bathroom and other doors.
- Make sure it's obvious which tap is hot and which is cold.
- Use non-slip mats.
- Fit locks that allow you to open the door from the outside in case your relative locks themselves inside.

Kitchens can be confusing and potentially dangerous – it is essential to your relative's independence and well-being to be able to navigate, understand and use the kitchen environment. Memory issues can make it difficult for your relative to remember what is behind each cupboard door.

- Leave frequently used items such as mugs, tea, coffee, spoons etc. on the countertop.
- Consider replacing solid doors with a see-through material such as glass or Perspex. Alternatively, you can remove doors completely or label each door with an image of what is inside.
- Make sure it is clear which tap is hot and which is cold – use waterproof labels if necessary.
- Keep on top of use-by dates and dump out-of-date food regularly to make sure your relative doesn't consume food that could make them ill.
- As the disease progresses, it may help to place simple instructions for using appliances next to each appliance.
- Keep toxic products out of reach or in a locked cupboard.
- Replace pots and pans with metal handles, which can become very hot, with those that have silicone, wood or bakelite.

Live well with assistive technology

Assistive technology incorporates devices or systems that help maintain or improve your relative's ability to perform everyday tasks. They can range from electronic pill boxes to smart home systems and include smartphone and tablet apps.

Equipment doesn't have to be massively expensive or complicated to help your relative live well with dementia. Some simple, inexpensive tools like a long-handled sponge or a pot with an easy-to-grip handle can make a huge difference to your relative's life. Everyone is different; what works for some may not work for others. It's helpful to contact dementia support services for more detailed, personalised advice that will take account of your relative's needs and preferences.

Assistive technology can significantly improve the quality of life for people with dementia by aiding memory, ensuring safety, supporting enjoyment and helping mobility. It can also help eliminate stress and make life a bit easier for you. Technology can be costly to buy new, so I'd recommend you google or ask your local Citizens Advice or support groups about renting technology or buying second-hand. Choose technology that is user-friendly and meets specific needs. And remember always to obtain consent from the person with dementia before implementing any technology. It's important to consider future needs and plan accordingly. You may be advised to introduce new technology or equipment earlier than it is needed while your relative retains the capacity to learn how to use it. Any technology you choose should enhance your relative's independence and fit well into your life and existing routines. Assistive technology should improve your life, so make sure that any tech you choose doesn't make your life more burdensome.

What you can do

Professional advice can help in selecting the most appropriate solutions. Discuss your relative's needs and abilities with your GP or an occupational therapist. They may help you to determine:

- If your relative needs technological support or whether there is another way to better support them.
- If the technology meets your relative's specific needs.
- Whether your relative has the cognitive ability to use the device.
- Whether your relative has the dexterity and can see and hear well enough to use the device.

- Whether the device needs ongoing technical support and maintenance.
- What the connectivity requirements are.
- What the full costs of purchasing and running the device are.

Make use of any local dementia centres where you can receive advice and try out devices.

Below are examples of some basic equipment and supportive technology that can help you both to live well.

Memory aids

- Whiteboards for lists and reminders.
- Calendars and diaries to keep track of appointments and routines.
- Clocks with easy-to-read numerals that also show the date.
- Talking clocks.
- Pill boxes with compartments for each day of the week can help your relative in the early to moderate stages of dementia keep track of medications.
- Automatic pill dispensers may be more appropriate for people in the late stages.

Many modern pill dispensers are designed to automatically dispense the correct medication at the right time and on the right day, helping people take their medications safely and accurately. Here's how they typically work:

- **Medication set-up:** You or your pharmacist load the dispenser with the correct pills, organised by day and time (e.g. morning, afternoon, evening doses). This is a great task to delegate to the pharmacist. Some devices allow for a week's supply, while others can hold medications for up to a month.
- **Programming:** The dispenser is set with the scheduled times for each dose. When the time comes, the dispenser will release the appropriate compartment with the correct medication.
- **Alerts and notifications:** When it's time to take medication, the dispenser typically sounds an alarm, flashes lights, or even sends

reminders via smartphone apps, depending on the device. Some dispensers will continue to alert until the pills are taken.
- **Automatic dispensing:** For fully automated dispensers, the device will release only the medication for the specific time. This prevents the user from accidentally taking the wrong pills or an incorrect dose.
- **Security features:** Many automatic dispensers are designed to prevent access to other compartments, so only the correct dose is accessible at any given time. This is particularly useful if your relative struggles with remembering or resisting the temptation to take more medication.
- **Missed dose handling:** Some advanced dispensers will track if a dose was missed and may alert you through an app.

Automated prompts and reminders

- **Devices that play set reminders:** You could record reminders for your relative that play at set times, for example reminding your relative to take their medication or to drink fluids.
- **Devices that detect motion:** There are a variety of devices that you can personalise to your relative's needs. For example, you could place a sensor or pressure mat at the exit from the kitchen that plays a message reminding your relative to switch off taps, hotplates, etc. before leaving the room.

While motion-sensing devices can be helpful, careful consideration and testing are essential to ensure they are beneficial and not potentially confusing for your relative, who may struggle with understanding sudden sounds or instructions coming from an unexpected source. They may not fully understand the purpose of the reminder or remember why they need to respond, especially if it's not immediately obvious where the voice is coming from. Unexpected sounds or messages might startle your relative, particularly if they aren't familiar with the device or if it's loud. Even if they understand the message initially, they may quickly forget to act on it by the time they get to the taps or hotplates. If the device activates frequently, it might lead to repeated confusion, frustration or anxiety, as they may not remember why the reminder keeps playing.

To reduce the risk of confusing or startling your relative, you could test the device to ensure the message is clear and calming. Use familiar voice prompts if possible (such as a family member's voice). Pair it with other support systems, like simple visual cues (for example, reminder signs near the taps or hotplates).

- **Smart devices:** There are numerous devices that will allow you to access devices in the home when you are not there, for example one that allows you to adjust the thermostat remotely.
- **Talking tiles:** You or your relative can record a message with the steps required to achieve things that will help your relative to maintain their independence despite memory issues. For example, one tile could have instructions for making a cup of tea, another for using the coffee machine, another for the washing machine or turning on the TV – basically, anything your relative would like to do that can be explained in a series of simple steps.

Some people may experience challenges completing a routine task like loading the dishwasher. A 'talking tile' allows you to record a message with the steps in a task. You place the tile where you need it – for example, beside the dishwasher. When your relative needs a prompt, they press the tile to hear the message.

- Locator devices designed for use by people with dementia tend to have a simple remote or base station that can trigger beeping sounds or flashing lights directly on the tagged item.
- Amazon Alexa and Google Assistant can answer questions posed by you or your relative. They can be useful for independence because your relative can ask questions such as 'Will I need a coat today?' or 'What day is it today?'

On the more expensive end of the scale are things like smart robots that can bring things to the person with dementia, vacuum the floor and remind your relative to take their keys when they leave the house. Robots are no substitute for humans and the care they provide. They should never be trusted implicitly but nonetheless have the potential to support you in your role as care partner.

Safety

There are many sensors and devices that closely monitor the whereabouts, movements and activities of a person with dementia. Monitoring and surveillance devices can provide valuable support in ensuring the safety of individuals with dementia, particularly for responding quickly in emergencies. However, it is crucial to approach their use with respect for the individual's autonomy and dignity. These devices should only be implemented with the informed and meaningful consent of the person with dementia, provided they have the capacity to understand and agree. If consent cannot be obtained due to diminished capacity, decisions should try to balance the individual's well-being with their right to privacy and autonomy. Best to involve family members and/or legal representatives, adhering to ethical and legal guidelines. These devices were developed to keep people safe; however, they can also be seen in a *Big Brother* way – as surveillance technology. If possible, discuss the potential use of such devices with your relative early on, and encourage them to record their decision on whether they would like to be monitored or not. Be sure your relative truly understands the full implications of using such devices.

Surveillance devices might include:

- **GPS trackers:** Devices that help care partners locate their relative if they leave their home or become lost. These generally come as wearable items like watches, pendants, or shoe inserts.
- **Video monitoring systems:** Cameras placed in common areas of the home to monitor activities remotely, ensuring your relative's safety without constant physical supervision.
- **Door and window sensors:** Sensors that alert care partners if a door or window is opened.
- **Motion sensors:** Devices that detect movement in specific areas, such as when your relative gets out of bed or moves around at unusual times.

- **Personal Emergency Response Systems (PERS):** Wearable devices with a button to call for help in case of emergencies such as falls or feeling lost or confused
- **Smart home devices:** Systems like Alexa or Google Home can assist with reminders and provide two-way communication while allowing remote monitoring through linked apps.
- **Medication dispensers with alerts:** Devices that notify care partners if medication has not been taken on time, often with integrated alarms or text alerts.
- **Bed or chair alarms:** Sensors placed under mattresses or on chairs that alert care partner if their relative moves unexpectedly, reducing the risk of falls.
- **Detection alarms:** Systems designed to alert care partners when their relative leaves a designated safe zone or crosses agreed set boundaries.
- **Two-way audio monitors:** Simple audio systems used for listening to your relative's activity or enabling easy communication between rooms in the same dwellings.

While these devices can enhance safety, they must be used responsibly and ethically, ensuring they align with your relative's rights and comfort.

Safety devices might include:

- Automatic lights with movement sensors that light the way to the bathroom at night or that come on automatically should your relative step out into the garden in darkness.
- Automatic shut-off devices for cookers that can turn off the gas supply or electricity before a fire starts.
- A kettle tipper that allows boiling water to be poured more safely.
- Water isolation devices that can automatically turn off taps to prevent flooding.
- Thermostat to control the temperature of water from kitchen taps.
- Timers to keep track of cooking time.

- Bath or sink plugs that open when water reaches a pre-set depth in the bath or sink.
- Scald prevention plugs for sinks and baths that change colour when the water gets too hot, to prevent burns.
- Long-handled sponges to make washing easier in the bath.
- A raised toilet seat.

Enjoyment

There are many tools and approaches that can help you and your relative live well and maintain a good quality of life. From adapting everyday devices to exploring helpful apps, small changes can make daily activities more enjoyable and accessible. Additionally, focusing on general health is essential for both of you. Here are some practical steps and resources to help you maintain physical, mental and emotional well-being.

Using a smartphone or tablet can open up many enjoyable and helpful activities for people with dementia, but it's important to remember that they may need some familiarity and confidence with the device first. Not all devices are equally easy to use, especially for those who may struggle with complex menus or small touchscreens.

There are several smartphones and tablets on the market designed to be simpler and more user-friendly. For example:

- GrandPad: This tablet is specifically designed for seniors, with large buttons, simplified menus and easy access to essential apps. It also features a support line for help.
- iPad: With its large screen and intuitive interface, the iPad can be a good option, especially if customised for simplicity.
- Jitterbug Smart3: This smartphone has a simple menu and larger icons, designed to be easier to navigate.

There are also some things you can do to make them easier to use. If your relative is already using a standard smartphone or tablet, you can make some adjustments to improve accessibility. You could place commonly used apps on a single home screen, grouping them in easy-to-identify folders (for example, 'Music', 'Videos', 'Calls') or with large, clear icons. Remove unnecessary apps or distractions so only essential apps are visible. This reduces the risk of confusion. Adjust settings for higher contrast and larger text to make it easier to read and navigate. Notifications can be overwhelming or confusing, so consider turning off non-essential alerts to keep the experience calm and straightforward. Many devices allow voice commands (like Siri on iPads or Google Assistant on Android). This can help users navigate without needing to type. If they need to learn how to use an app, try providing simple step-by-step instructions or create a visual guide they can refer to. Supporting your relative with dementia in using a smartphone or tablet can empower them to stay connected, entertained and engaged in a way that feels manageable and enjoyable. With the right adjustments and encouragement, these devices can become a valuable part of their daily routine.

Adapt: Everyday technology and household equipment adapted for people with dementia (e.g. single knob radios, remote controls and mobile phones with simplified buttons) so that they can continue to enjoy using them.

Apps: There is a multitude of apps available that can help you and your relative to continue to enjoy life and live well:

- Listen to music
- Watch videos
- Video-call friends and family
- Arrange and coordinate caregiving activities
- Meditation or mindfulness apps to help with relaxation and stress management
- To-do list apps
- Reminder calendar apps
- Singalong apps
- Dance apps
- Yoga apps
- Physical exercise apps
- Speech therapy apps
- Falls prevention apps
- Games and puzzles apps

The list is constantly growing and practically endless.

Live well in good health

Section 1 contains a great deal of information that will help you as the care partner to live well in good health while you care for your relative with dementia. It is important also to look after your relative's general health. It is all too easy for dementia to take over, as if that is the only issue that can interfere with health and enjoyment of life in later years.

What you can do

Dementia can be so all-consuming, it is easy to neglect other aspects of health. Make sure both you and your relative do the following:

- Get your vision and eye health tested regularly.
- Get your vaccinations (flu, Covid, etc.).
- Go for regular GP check-ups.
- Get your hearing tested regularly.
- Visit the dentist for regular cleaning and check-ups.
- Get your blood pressure tested regularly.

Brain health

Looking after brain health is critical for everyone, including those already diagnosed with dementia. Our brain is our most important organ, yet most of us rarely give it a second thought. What you do or don't do influences how well your brain functions now and how resilient it can be when faced with future challenges. This flexibility is called neuroplasticity and allows you to learn new things and adapt to changes in your life and in your environment at any age. Neuroplasticity underlies resilience and is critical to brain health.

Adopting a brain-healthy lifestyle is like investing in brain capital because it not only helps you to optimise brain function now, it also allows you to build cognitive reserves that can be cashed in at some point in the future to cope with or compensate for brain disease, damage or age-related decline in cognitive function. Adopting a brain-healthy approach to life may help to prevent or slow down the rate at which your brain shrinks with age or dementia.

Below you will find numerous ways to keep your brain healthy and reduce dementia risk, broken down into three categories: activity, lifestyle and attitude.

Activity

Physical exercise, social engagement and mental activity are all essential to brain health.

Physical exercise

Exercise is already covered in section 1, but I want to share a few insights with you that might motivate you to get physically active. Most people are surprised to learn that physical exercise is one of the best things they can do for their brain health. The brain is a high-energy organ that needs a healthy and constant supply of oxygen. Exercise helps to maintain the blood flow and the supply of oxygen and nutrients to the brain. Healthy blood flow reduces risk for cardiovascular disease and stroke, which increase a person's risk factors for dementia. Physical activity also helps to reduce the brain's exposure to neurotoxins including beta-amyloid, a build-up of which is implicated in Alzheimer's disease. Neurochemicals are released when we exercise that promote the growth of new brain cells and connections in a part of the brain that plays a critical role in learning and memory.

Physical inactivity is a risk factor for dementia that is also associated with other dementia risk factors including diabetes, depression and high blood pressure. About four million cases of Alzheimer's disease around the globe are potentially attributable to physical inactivity. Physical inactivity accelerates the ageing process while physical activity slows it down. Prolonged periods of sitting slow down metabolism, affecting the body's ability to regulate blood pressure and blood sugar and break down body fat. Exercise and a healthy diet don't just allow you to live longer, they allow you to live better.

What you can do

Exercise daily – even 10 minutes is beneficial. Sit less. Stand more. Straighten up. Move more. Swap screen time for physical activity.

Here are some enjoyable and innovative ways for you and your relative to integrate more physical exercise into daily life. These activities focus on keeping things light-hearted, engaging and suitable for various ability levels.

> **GENERAL TIPS**
>
> - **Focus on fun, not fitness:** Emphasise the enjoyment of the activity rather than the exercise aspect. This reduces pressure and encourages engagement.
> - **Incorporate routines:** Try to make these activities a regular part of the day or week, so they feel natural and not like a workout.
> - **Adapt and be flexible:** Be mindful of energy levels and mood, adapting the intensity and duration to what feels comfortable and enjoyable.

- Dancing is a fantastic way to get moving without it feeling like exercise. Play music from your relative's youth or a song you used to dance to together as a couple. This can stimulate positive memories and make your relative more likely to engage. Try different styles – from slow waltzes to fun line dances. You can even turn it into a daily dance break (not break dance) routine. Experiment till you find something that works that you both enjoy. Dancing improves balance, enhances mood and can be done at home with minimal set-up.
- Make walking more purposeful by creating small 'missions' or themes. For example, have a 'nature walk' where you look for certain flowers or animals, or a 'photo walk' where you take photos of interesting things you find. Parks and gardens are great places for this. This kind of walking provides light cardio, adds cognitive engagement and encourages exploration.

- If mobility is limited, seated exercises can be a great option. There are fun online classes tailored to older adults that include chair-based routines set to music, or you can create your own with movements like arm raises, gentle leg lifts and stretching. Chair exercises build strength, improve flexibility and can be done together at home.
- Gardening is a wonderful physical activity that involves squatting, bending, lifting and fine motor skills. If you have space outdoors, light weeding, planting or watering can be enjoyable. Gardening enhances flexibility, provides sensory stimulation and allows for a calming connection with nature.
- Games like balloon volleyball or gentle table tennis are fun and adaptable to all ability levels. These can be done indoors with minimal equipment – a balloon or soft beach ball for volleyball, or a foam ball and paddles on the kitchen table for table tennis.
- Games such as these improve hand-eye coordination, encourage social interaction and bring in light cardio.
- Yoga or tai chi, adapted for seniors, can be done at home or in a local class. Both are low impact and gentle, focusing on stretching, balance and breathing. Look for simple routines you can follow together, either online or in a group setting. These practices enhance flexibility, improve balance and promote relaxation.
- Turn chores into an activity you do together. Simple tasks like folding laundry, sweeping or light dusting can provide movement and a sense of accomplishment. To make it more enjoyable, try setting a timer and challenging each other to see how much you can do in five minutes. This type of movement makes the home environment pleasant and provides a sense of purpose.
- Many communities offer walking groups or outdoor classes designed for seniors. Joining these can provide social interaction and create a regular routine. Some classes may include strength training, stretching or mobility exercises in a relaxed group environment, which builds social connections, improves fitness and offers variety.

These ideas blend physical activity with social, sensory and cognitive engagement, helping both you and your relative to stay active in ways that bring enjoyment and connection.

Social engagement

As a care partner, you are at risk for becoming socially isolated and lonely. I think it's worthwhile outlining more of the science behind why you need to prioritise it in your life. The dementia risk associated with loneliness and social isolation is comparable in size with well-known risk factors for Alzheimer's disease including physical inactivity, mid-life high blood pressure, type 2 diabetes, smoking and depression. People with more social ties are less likely to develop dementia or a cognitive impairment.

It is critical that you take action to ensure your life and the life of your relative are socially integrated. It's all too easy to lock yourselves away from the world while dementia takes centre stage. Seek out opportunities for social engagement where you can; there is no point in increasing your own risk of developing the disease while you care for your relative.

Social connection will benefit your relative too, because living a life that is socially integrated and engaged is associated with slower cognitive decline. Social interactions bring about structural and functional plastic changes in the brain. Socially engaged lifestyles and stimulating environments are associated with the growth of new neurons and an increase in the density of connections. Social activity increases brain volume and leads to more efficient use of brain networks.

What you can do

If you have already become a bit isolated, it can be hard to take action to re-engage. Start small. Make time for social activities. Get out and about – a walk in the park or a trip to the shops can offer opportunities for a chat. Participate in groups for people living with dementia and their care partners – while this might seem like a busman's holiday initially, it really can become a social outlet for care partners. Of course, initial conversations on joining will be about your relative, but if you stick with it you will find other interests in common and may build new friendships.

Attend events that welcome people with dementia. Schedule regular phone or video conversations with family and friends. Join online groups. Take classes locally or online.

Mental activity

Remember the old adage: 'Use it or lose it!' As you age, neurons that are left out of action through lack of use become damaged and die. Engaging the brain in stimulating leisure activities may allow people to cope with Alzheimer's brain changes for longer before manifesting memory loss. Stimulation doesn't prevent your brain from becoming diseased, but it does seem to lessen the impact that the disease has on cognitive functioning.

Challenging your brain promotes neuroplasticity. Novelty – experiencing new things, new people and new situations – is a critical element of neuroplasticity. Lifelong learning also results in reduced risk of social isolation. Learning is like a powerful brain-changing drug that generates new brain cells, enriches brain networks and opens new routes that the brain can use to bypass damage. Below are some general suggestions for activities that are mentally stimulating – but before you despair and think I'm going to tell you to learn Spanish, remember that your journey as a care partner is paved with opportunities for mental stimulation. You are constantly learning new things and new ways of doing old things. You have to learn to navigate new systems and jump through administrative hoops. Reframe these things as opportunities to keep your brain healthy rather than stress-inducing challenges that you have to overcome.

What you can do

Embrace the changes in your life now and reimagine them as opportunities to boost your brain health. Remember, social engagement is a form of mental stimulation. You could join a book club (it can be virtual) or take courses that interest you (they can be online). Learn how the assistive technology for your relative works. You could get involved in dementia advocacy. Reconnect with hobbies you may have dropped. If, for example, you played an instrument in the past, start playing again; or if you still play, add a more challenging piece to your repertoire. You can apply this approach to almost any hobby or pastime – it doesn't matter whether it's wood-turning or knitting, the principle is the same. Set yourself challenges, learn new things, push yourself beyond your comfort zone.

Lifestyle

Sleep

I've already made the case for prioritising sleep in section 1, so look back for some ideas to help you sleep well. But if you are not yet convinced, here is some additional information. Sleep is critical for clearing the brain of toxins, including those involved in Alzheimer's disease. Sleep is essential for learning, memory and attention. Sleep deprivation interferes with neuroplasticity, which is critical for brain health and resilience. Your brain needs both non-REM and REM sleep so get your sleep at the right time, preferably beginning between eight and midnight. New information is strengthened and new memories are consolidated during non-REM sleep. New information is integrated with existing information, experiences and memories during REM sleep, allowing you to problem-solve, gain insight and develop ideas. As we get older, we don't need less sleep but we may experience decline in the quantity, quality and efficiency of our sleep and may need to go to bed earlier than we did in the past to compensate. The only thing that can relieve sleep pressure and rid your system of the sleep pressure chemical is sleep.

Driving while drowsy can be as dangerous as driving under the influence of alcohol.

Sleep deprivation also leads to weight gain. Research shows that just one week of sleep deprivation can send you into a pre-diabetic state.

What you can do

Make sleep a priority by following the advice in section 1. Make a point to avoid caffeine and alcohol close to bedtime. Doing some physical activity during the day will also help.

Heart health

Your brain is highly dependent on your heart and your blood vessels to deliver the oxygen and nutrients essential for the functioning and survival of your brain cells.

Damage to this vascular system can have catastrophic consequences for you and for your brain. About a third of all cases of dementia can be attributed to vascular issues.

Blood pressure is particularly important for brain health. High blood pressure can cause damage to your arteries and your heart and over time this can disrupt the delivery of vital supplies to your brain. Stroke and the factors that lead to it play a pivotal role in cognitive impairment and dementia.

When it comes to heart health and brain health, maintaining a healthy diet is key. What you eat directly affects your brain function and its structure. Your brain is incredibly vulnerable and highly dependent on you to provide it with the fuel, water, nutrients and oxygen that it needs to function. If you become deficient in omega 3, you will likely experience memory problems. A vitamin B12 deficiency, which can be easily treated, can look a lot like dementia. Chronic dehydration can increase your risk of high blood pressure and stroke. Diets that are high in sugars promote oxidative stress, which can lead to heart and blood vessel disorders and neurodegenerative diseases. Eating a balanced diet rich in vitamins, minerals and antioxidants can protect your brain from oxidative stress.

In addition to impacting on cardiovascular health smoking also kills brain cells. The cortex is the outer layer of the brain responsible for critical functions like memory, attention and solving problems. Smokers have thinner cortices than non-smokers. The longer you smoke, the thinner your cortex gets. When the cortex becomes thinner, it can lead to a decline in cognitive abilities, making it harder to think clearly, remember information and process complex tasks.

What you can do

In addition to the advice in section 1 about adopting the Mediterranean diet, there are a few other simple things you can try. First, be kind to your brain and eat regularly and stay hydrated. Get in the habit of reading food labels, make more informed choices, go easy on the sugar, skip the salt, increase your water intake and reduce alcohol consumption.

Hearing

Age-related hearing loss is one of the biggest risk factors for dementia. Thankfully, you can mitigate this risk by getting your hearing checked regularly, avoiding exposure to loud noises and wearing hearing aids if prescribed. Untreated hearing loss also impacts on the quality of your life and can lead to depression, unhealthy coping behaviours and a self-imposed social isolation.

What you can do

Protect your ears from excessive noise, and wear ear defenders if you are near or use noisy machinery or have a job where loud music is played. Reduce the volume on your headphones. Get your hearing tested annually. Wear hearing aids if they are prescribed.

Attitude

Stress

The stress response is neither good nor bad, it simply evolved and still exists to support your survival, which it does extremely well in acute situations. However, as you learned in section 1, stress becomes problematic when it is prolonged or poorly managed. Stress steals resources that would be better used in other ways.

What you can do

Commit to following the advice on managing stress in section 1. Remember that taking regular exercise, prioritising sleep, socialising and having fun are all great ways to manage stress.

Smile

Smiling boosts brain health. Smiling makes your brain more flexible, more resilient and better able to cope with life's challenges. Smiling releases hormones that make you feel good, lowers blood pressure, boosts immune function and protects against stress, depression and anxiety.

What you can do

Start and end your day with a smile and in between make sure you smile at least five times, even – or especially – if you don't feel like it. It's amazing but true, as research has shown, that the simple act of smiling sends messages to your brain that can make you happy even if you are not. Share at least one smile with someone else. It's contagious and can lead to laughter. Spread the happiness and the health benefits.

Gratitude

We know that regular practice of gratitude can enhance our psychological well-being. People who practise gratitude derive more pleasure and happiness from everyday life. While the effects of gratitude are not instant, with time and practice they impact positively on our physical and psychological health. Gratitude is a powerful human emotion. Writing detailed, heartfelt notes to people who have positively influenced your life elicits feelings of contentment. Gratitude increases self-satisfaction, improves mood and enhances positive emotions and thoughts. Gratitude is linked with increased vitality and energy. Gratitude bolsters happiness and induces contentment and pleasure.

Keeping a gratitude journal can lower your stress levels, improve sleep quality and even alleviate pain. Regularly expressing gratitude genuinely mitigates against stress and anxiety. Practising gratitude can retrain your brain to prioritise positivity and help you accept life's uncertainties and feel less fearful about the future. Practising gratitude daily can potentially have effects akin to antidepressants, providing a sense of long-lasting happiness and contentment.

From a neuroscience perspective, gratitude activates the brain's bliss centres. When you regularly express gratitude, it stimulates the release of serotonin and dopamine, which are associated with feelings of pleasure, reward, motivation, satisfaction, happiness and optimism.

GRATITUDE

Máire-Anne

'Some days didn't go as well as others during my time caring for my dad (in fact, there were some days I felt I was not a good carer, I wasn't even a good daughter), and of course the guilt at night almost smothered me – until I spoke to a friend who had cared for her father (who had Parkinson's and dementia). It was while we were chatting that the subject came up casually. She mentioned what she would do at the end of every day before her dad went to sleep – she would tell him how much she loved him and thank him for the day they had together. From that day forward, I did exactly that, and every night Dad's reaction was always the same: 'Aw, that is lovely, and I love you too, sweetheart.' And being the gorgeous dad he was, he always added that he looked forward to spending the next day with me. I headed to bed with a HUGE smile on my face, knowing Dad was content and probably still smiling, and I slept like a baby knowing that that particular day was filed away/complete, and I too looked forward to a new day with my dad.

What you can do

Dementia can blind us to the simple pleasures of life. The shadows cast by this spectre can fool us into thinking that there is nothing in our lives but bleakness and loss. But that is not true. Dementia steals many things, but it does not take away the simple pleasures of life. There are many, many things that remain within our gift that we can be grateful for. We can still love and be loved. The present moment remains ours to enjoy. We can be kind. We can dance. We can sing. We can laugh. We can cry. We can hug and be hugged. We can hold hands. We can offer and receive solace. We can feel joy, experience pleasure and appreciate beauty. We can taste food, savour scents, and share a sunset. Keep a gratitude journal and reap the benefits.

All is not lost. Care for yourself and be grateful for and treasure what remains.

Section 3 – Summary

Key messages

- People with dementia want a good quality of life, they want to do as much for themselves as possible and they still want to have fun and experience pleasure.
- Cognitive stimulation therapy (CST), which is delivered in a group setting, improves quality of life, memory and thinking skills in people with mild to moderate dementia.
- Research shows that the benefits of CST are equivalent to a six-month delay in expected cognitive decline in people with mild to moderate dementia.
- Improvements in communication, quality of life, mood and depression are reported, as well as reduction in aggression and 'caregiver burden'.
- CST offers people with dementia a sense of purpose and opportunities to socialise and share their experience with others.
- Cognitive rehabilitation aims to make everyday life easier for people living with mild to moderate dementia by helping them with some of the changes that dementia can bring.
- Cognitive rehabilitation is a personalised therapy that aims to help individuals to function as well as possible, engage in meaningful activities and maintain their independence.
- Cognitive rehabilitation involves setting personal goals and identifying areas of functioning that the person with dementia would like to improve and which are important to them.
- Having goals enriches life, giving it purpose and meaning. This is something that applies to all of us, including those living with dementia and their care partners.
- Simple changes can make big differences. Small wins accumulate and can add up to big changes in mood and quality of life.
- Behavioural and psychological symptoms in dementia (BPSD) are common and often cause the most stress and burden in care partners.

- Neuropsychiatric symptoms can be upsetting and physically and mentally exhausting.
- Your relative may only occasionally experience neuropsychiatric symptoms or their symptoms may be mild or relatively easy to manage.
- Living well with dementia involves a combination of self-care, practical planning, maintaining health, creating a supportive environment with a focus on your relative and on positive experiences.
- Dementia can make it difficult for a person affected to recognise where they are or what time of day it is.

Practical tips

- It's important that you try and maintain outside activities if possible, so that you have connections and opportunities when your caring journey ends.
- Set yourself goals that will provide you with personal satisfaction outside of your caregiving role. Keep them small and specific.
- Use the questions on page 193 of Chapter 9 to help your relative identify small goals that can make a significant difference to their quality of life. Consider asking yourself the same questions.
- Ask your GP whether CST or cognitive rehabilitation is available in your area and if so ask them to write a referral if you think these interventions would be of benefit.
- Communicate with your relative with empathy and understanding, speak in a calm, loving voice, maintain eye contact and use gentle touch.
- Set up routines: they will minimise your stress and may be soothing for your relative.
- Use music, aromas and touch where appropriate to soothe your relative.
- Avoid over stimulating your relative, remove clutter or ask someone to help you to declutter.
- Get yourself and your relative out in daylight and nature as often as you can.

- Encourage and enjoy physical exercise, healthy diet and fun activities.
- Use this book and this section in particular as a resource to help you understand, manage and minimise neuropsychiatric symptoms.
- Problems that are ignored or avoided don't usually resolve on their own and can become more significant or complicated.
- Adopt coping strategies that involve problem-solving, support, meditation or mindfulness and physical exercise.
- Anxiety is best managed through engagement and activity in the first instance.
- Systematically observing, recording and interpreting your relative's behaviour will help you to identify triggers and unmet needs, making life more manageable for both of you.
- Shifting your focus away from the disease to your relative and the present will help you to continue enjoying life, despite dementia.
- Encourage your relative to record their preferences and wishes as soon as possible after diagnosis. Having clearly articulated preferences and wishes will reduce stress for everyone involved and will limit family arguments and emotional upheaval.
- Manipulating light will help orient your relative to time and prevent confusion.
- Make it easier for your relative to navigate their home by using colour contrast to define the environment.
- Small modifications to various rooms in your relative's home can help them to remain independent for longer.
- Basic equipment can support your relative to perform everyday tasks.
- Assistive technology can significantly improve the quality of life for your relative by aiding memory, ensuring safety, supporting enjoyment and helping mobility.
- Always obtain consent from your relative before implementing any technology.
- Never employ a surveillance or monitoring device without your relative's explicit consent. Be sure your relative truly understands the full implications of using such devices.

- Dementia doesn't offer immunity to other conditions that are common in later life. It is critical to continue regular health checks.
- Adopt brain healthy habits for your relative and yourself. Looking after brain health is critical for everyone, including those already diagnosed with dementia and their care partner.
- Understand dementia, then focus on your relative rather than the disease. Care for yourself and be grateful for and treasure what remains.

Appendix

Care partner diary activities

1. Caregiving	
Personal care	Assistance with: showering, bathing, dressing, hair washing, shaving, brushing teeth, brushing/combing hair, applying make-up, applying non-medical skin care, nail care, etc.
Toileting	Assistance with: getting to and from the bathroom, assistance on to toilet/commode, bedpan, incontinence care, etc.
Mobility	Assistance with: walking, rising from and getting into chair/bed, turning in bed, home exercises (physical activity, range of motion exercises), etc.
Nutrition	Preparing meals and snacks, assisting with eating, feeding, preparation and provision of fluids, monitoring and managing fluid intake, preparing 'soft' food and thickening drinks, etc.
Support	Laundry, buying clothes, washing dishes, keeping bedroom and bathroom clean.
Medical	Filling prescriptions, picking up prescriptions, filling weekly pill organiser, giving medication, ensuring medication is taken, scheduling medical appointments, accompanying to medical appointments, monitoring symptoms, communicating with healthcare professionals, advocating for supports and services, etc.
Companionship	Engaging with your relative in the following ways: chatting, reading aloud, listening to music, singing, playing games, painting, providing verbal and non-verbal emotional support, going for walks together, socialising together, watching TV, going on trips together, etc.
Supervision	Ensuring your relative's safety during the day and throughout the night, for example when walking, going to the bathroom or carrying out tasks such as cooking.
Transport	To medical appointments, to respite, to social and religious activities, etc.
Other	

References

1. Burden

Cheng, S.T. (2017). "Dementia caregiver burden: a research update and critical analysis." *Current Psychiatry Reports, 19*(9), 64. https://doi.org/10.1007/s11920-017-0818-2

Gräßel, E. (1990). *Pflegeabhängigkeit und Belastung: Ein sozialgerontologisches Modell zur Früherkennung von Risikofamilien.* Dissertation, University of Erlangen-Nuremberg, Germany.

Gräßel, E., Chiu, T., & Oliver, R. (2003). Development and validation of the Burden Scale for Family Caregivers (BSFC). *COTA Comprehensive Rehabilitation and Mental Health Services*, Toronto, Ontario, Canada.

Moniz-Cook, E., et al. (2008). "A European consensus on outcome measures for psychosocial intervention research in dementia care." *Aging & Mental Health, 12*(1), 14–29.

Olsen, C., Pedersen, I., Bergland, A., et al. (2016). "Differences in quality of life in home-dwelling persons and nursing home residents with dementia – a cross-sectional study." *BMC Geriatrics, 16*, 137. https://doi.org/10.1186/s12877-016-0312-4

Pinquart, M., & Sörensen, S. (2003). "Associations of stressors and uplifts of caregiving with caregiver burden and depressive mood: a meta-analysis." *Journal of Gerontology: Series B, Psychological Sciences and Social Sciences, 58*(2), 112–128.

2. Health

Andre, C.J., Lovallo, V., & Spencer, R.M.C. (2021). "The effects of bed sharing on sleep: From partners to pets." *Sleep Health, 7*(3), 314–323.

Brodaty, H., & Donkin, M. (2009). "Family caregivers of people with dementia." *Dialogues in Clinical Neuroscience, 11*(2), 217–228.

Dias, R., et al. (2015). "Resilience of caregivers of people with dementia: a systematic review of biological and psychosocial determinants." *Trends in Psychiatry and Psychotherapy, 37*(1), 12–19. https://doi.org/10.1590/2237-6089-2014-0032

Drews, H.J., Wallot, S., Brysch, P., et al. (2020). "Bed-sharing in couples is associated with increased and stabilized REM sleep and sleep-stage synchronization." *Frontiers in Psychiatry, 11*. https://doi.org/10.3389/fpsyt.2020.00583

Gao, C., et al. (2019). "Sleep duration and sleep quality in caregivers of patients with dementia: A systematic review and meta-analysis." *JAMA Network Open, 2*(8), e199891. https://doi.org/10.1001/jamanetworkopen.2019.9891

Hanlon, E.C., Tasali, E., Leproult, R., Stuhr, K.L., Doncheck, E., de Wit, H., Hillard, C.J., & Van Cauter, E. (2016). "Sleep restriction enhances the daily rhythm of circulating levels of endocannabinoid 2-arachidonoylglycerol." *Sleep, 39*(3), 653–664. https://doi.org/10.5665/sleep.5546

Harmell, A.L., et al. (2011). "A review of the psychobiology of dementia caregiving: A focus on resilience factors." *Current Psychiatry Reports, 13*(3), 219–224.

Hann, D., Winter, K., & Jacobsen, P. (1999). "Measurement of depressive symptoms in cancer patients: Evaluation of the Center for Epidemiological Studies Depression Scale (CES-D)." *Journal of Psychosomatic Research, 46*, 437–443.

Huang, S.S. (2022). "Depression among caregivers of patients with dementia: Associative factors and management approaches." *World Journal of Psychiatry, 12*(1), 59–76. https://doi.org/10.5498/wjp.v12.i1.59

Khatib, H.K.A., Harding, S.V., Darzi, J., & Pot, G.K. (2016). "The effects of partial sleep deprivation on energy balance: A systematic review and meta-analysis." *European Journal of Clinical Nutrition*. Published online November 2, 2016. https://doi.org/10.1038/ejcn.2016.201

Masud, H. (2021). "Sleep and neurodegenerative diseases." *Brain, 144*(3), 695–696. https://doi.org/10.1093/brain/awab031

Mattos, M.K., et al. (2024). "Sleep and caregiver burden among caregivers of persons living with dementia: A scoping review." *Innovation in Aging, 8*(2), igae005. https://doi.org/10.1093/geroni/igae005

Mayer-Suess, L., Ibrahim, A., Moelgg, K., et al. (2024). "Sleep disorders as both risk factors for, and a consequence of, stroke: A narrative review." *International Journal of Stroke, 19*(5), 490–498. https://doi.org/10.1177/17474930231212349

McCurry, S.M., et al. (2007). "Sleep disturbances in caregivers of persons with dementia: Contributing factors and treatment implications." *Sleep Medicine Reviews, 11*(2), 143–153. https://doi.org/10.1016/j.smrv.2006.09.002

Radloff, L.S. (1977). "The CES-D Scale: A self-report depression scale for research in the general population." *Applied Psychological Measurement, 1*, 385–401.

Schulz, R., & Sherwood, P.R. (2008). "Physical and mental health effects of family caregiving." *American Journal of Nursing, 108*(9 Suppl), 23–27.

Simpson, C., & Carter, P. (2015). "The impact of living arrangements on dementia caregivers' sleep quality." *American Journal of Alzheimer's Disease & Other Dementias, 30*(4), 352–359. https://doi.org/10.1177/1533317514559828

Song, M.J., & Kim, J.H. (2021). "Family caregivers of people with dementia have poor sleep quality: A nationwide population-based study." *International Journal of Environmental Research and Public Health, 18*(24), 13079. https://doi.org/10.3390/ijerph182413079

Taylor, K., Tripathi, A.K., & Jones, E.B. (2022). "Adult dehydration." *StatPearls [Internet]*. Treasure Island (FL): StatPearls Publishing.

Voderholzer, U., Al-Shajlawi, A., Weske, G., Feige, B., & Riemann, D. (2003). "Are there gender differences in objective and subjective sleep measures? A study of insomniacs and healthy controls." *Depression and Anxiety, 17*(3), 162–172. https://doi.org/10.1002/da.10101

Vitaliano, P.P., Zhang, J., & Scanlan, J.M. (2003). "Is caregiving hazardous to one's physical health? A meta-analysis." *Psychological Bulletin, 129*(6), 946–972. https://doi.org/10.1037/0033-2909.129.6.946

Vitaliano, P.P., et al. (2011). "Does caring for a spouse with dementia promote cognitive decline? A hypothesis and proposed mechanisms." *Journal of the American Geriatrics Society, 59*(5), 900–908.

Wennberg, A.M.V., Wu, M.N., Rosenberg, P.B., & Spira, A.P. (2017). "Sleep disturbance, cognitive decline, and dementia: A review." *Seminars in Neurology, 37*(4), 395–406. https://doi.org/10.1055/s-0037-1604351

Xu, W., Tan, C., Zou, J., et al. (2020). "Sleep problems and risk of all-cause cognitive decline or dementia: An updated systematic review and meta-analysis." *Journal of Neurology, Neurosurgery & Psychiatry, 91*, 236–244.

3. Stress

Brennan, S. (2021). *Beating Brain Fog: Your 30-Day Plan to Think Sharper, Faster, Better.* Orion Spring.

Brodaty, H., & Hadzi-Pavlovic, D. (1990). "Psychosocial effects on carers of living with persons with dementia." *Australian and New Zealand Journal of Psychiatry, 24*(3), 351–361. https://doi.org/10.3109/00048679009077702

Lovibond, S.H., & Lovibond, P.F. (1995). *Manual for the Depression Anxiety Stress Scales* (2nd ed.). Sydney: Psychology Foundation.

Ory, M., et al. (1999). "Prevalence and impact of caregiving: A detailed comparison between dementia and non-dementia care partners." *The Gerontologist, 39*, 177–185.

Pinquart, M., & Sörensen, S. (2003). "Differences between caregivers and non-caregivers in psychological health and physical health: A meta-analysis." *Psychology and Aging, 18*, 250–267.

Schulz, R., & Sherwood, P.R. (2008). "Physical and mental health effects of family caregiving." *American Journal of Nursing, 108*(9 Suppl), 23–27.

Vitaliano, P.P., et al. (2009). "Depressed mood mediates decline in cognitive processing speed in caregivers." *The Gerontologist, 49*(1), 12–22.

4. Support

Ditzen, B., & Heinrichs, M. (2014). "Psychobiology of social support: The social dimension of stress buffering." *Restorative Neurology and Neuroscience, 32*, 149–162. https://doi.org/10.3233/RNN-139008

Zimet, G.D., Dahlem, N.W., Zimet, S.G., & Farley, G.K. (1988). "The Multidimensional Scale of Perceived Social Support." *Journal of Personality Assessment, 52*(1), 30–41. https://doi.org/10.1207/s15327752jpa5201_2

5. Coping

Gilhooly, K.J., et al. (2016). "A meta-review of stress, coping, and interventions in dementia and dementia caregiving." *BMC Geriatrics, 18*(16), 106. https://doi.org/10.1186/s12877-016-0280-8

Iavarone, A., et al. (2014). "Caregiver burden and coping strategies in care partners of patients with Alzheimer's disease." *Neuropsychiatric Disease and Treatment, 10*, 1407–1413. https://doi.org/10.2147/NDT.S58063

Pearlin, L.I. (1989). "The sociological study of stress." *Journal of Health and Social Behavior, 30*, 241–256.

Pearlin, L.I. (1990). "Caregiving and the stress process: An overview of concepts and their measures." *The Gerontologist, 30*(5), 583–594.

Schulz, R., & Sherwood, P.R. (2008). "Physical and mental health effects of family caregiving." *American Journal of Nursing, 108*(9 Suppl), 23–27.

Snyder, C.M., et al. (2015). "Dementia caregivers' coping strategies and their relationship to health and well-being: The Cache County Study." *Aging & Mental Health, 19*(5), 390–399. https://doi.org/10.1080/13607863.2014.939610

6. Reward

Cheng, S.T. (2017). "Dementia caregiver burden: A research update and critical analysis." *Current Psychiatry Reports, 19*(9), 64. https://doi.org/10.1007/s11920-017-0818-2

Fredman, L., et al. (2015). "The relationship between caregiving and mortality after accounting for time-varying caregiver status and addressing the healthy caregiver hypothesis." *Journals of Gerontology: Medical Sciences, 70*(9), 1163–1168. https://doi.org/10.1093/gerona/glv009

7. See Me

Brown, M., et al. (2020). "Meaningful activity in advanced dementia." *Nursing Older People*. Published online September 2. https://doi.org/10.7748/nop.2020.e1171

Gebhard, D., & Frank, J.I. (2024). "Everyday life and boredom of people living with dementia in residential long-term care: A merged methods study." *BMC Geriatrics, 24*, 1049. https://doi.org/10.1186/s12877-024-05641-7

9. Making the most of what you've got

Bailey, J., et al. (2017). "An evaluation of Cognitive Stimulation Therapy sessions for people with dementia and a concomitant support group for their carers." *Dementia (London), 16*(8), 985–1003. https://doi.org/10.1177/1471301215626851

Clare, L., Kudlicka, A., Oyebode, J.R., Jones, R.W., Bayer, A., Leroi, I., Kopelman, M., James, I.A., Culverwell, A., Pool, J., Brand, A., Henderson, C., Hoare, Z., Knapp, M., Woods, B. (2019). "Individual goal-oriented cognitive rehabilitation to improve everyday functioning for people with early-stage dementia: A multicentre randomised controlled trial (the GREAT trial)." *International Journal of Geriatric Psychiatry, 34*(5), 709–721. https://doi.org/10.1002/gps.5076

Kudlicka, A., et al. (2019). "Cognitive rehabilitation for people with mild to moderate dementia." *Cochrane Database of Systematic Reviews.* https://doi.org/10.1002/14651858.CD013388

Kudlicka, A., Martyr, A., Bahar-Fuchs, A., Sabates, J., Woods, B., & Clare, L. (2023). "Cognitive rehabilitation for people with mild to moderate dementia." *Cochrane Database of Systematic Reviews, 2023*(6), CD013388. https://doi.org/10.1002/14651858.CD013388.pub2

Lobbia, A., et al. (2019). "The efficacy of Cognitive Stimulation Therapy (CST) for people with mild-to-moderate dementia: A review." *European Psychologist, 24*(3), 257–277. https://doi.org/10.1027/1016-9040/a000342

Saragih, I.D., et al. (2022). "Effects of Cognitive Stimulation Therapy for people with dementia: A systematic review and meta-analysis of randomized controlled studies." *International Journal of Nursing Studies, 128*, 104181. https://doi.org/10.1016/j.ijnurstu.2022.104181

Wehrmann, H., et al. (2021). "Priorities and preferences of people living with dementia or cognitive impairment – A systematic review." *Patient Preference and Adherence, 15*, 2793–2807. https://doi.org/10.2147/PPA.S333923

Woods, B., et al. (2023). "Cognitive stimulation to improve cognitive functioning in people with dementia." *Cochrane Database of Systematic Reviews, 2023*(1), CD005562. https://doi.org/10.1002/14651858.CD005562.pub3

10. Minimising the tough stuff

Ayalon, L., & Gum, A.M. (2011). "The relationships between major depression, neuropsychiatric symptoms, and quality of life in Alzheimer's disease." *Aging & Mental Health, 15*(8), 1063–1071.

Calsolaro, V., et al. (2021). "Behavioral and psychological symptoms in dementia (BPSD) and the use of antipsychotics." *Pharmaceuticals (Basel), 14*(3), 246. https://doi.org/10.3390/ph14030246

Cerejeira, J., et al. (2012). "Behavioral and psychological symptoms of dementia." *Frontiers in Neurology, 3*, 73. https://doi.org/10.3389/fneur.2012.00073

Cohen-Mansfield, J., et al. (1995). "Temporal patterns of agitation in nursing home residents with dementia." *Journal of Gerontology, 50*(6), P366–P373.

Costello, H., et al. (2023). "Antidepressant medications in dementia: Evidence and potential mechanisms of treatment resistance." *Psychological Medicine, 53*(3), 654–667. https://doi.org/10.1017/S003329172200397X

Cummings, J.L., & McPherson, S. (2001). "Neuropsychiatric assessment of Alzheimer's disease and related dementias." *Aging & Mental Health, 5*(1), 21–25.

El Haj, M., et al. (2017). "Clinical and neurocognitive aspects of hallucinations in Alzheimer's disease." *Neuroscience & Biobehavioral Reviews, 83*, 713–720. https://doi.org/10.1016/j.neurobiorev.2017.02.021

Gauthier, S., et al. (2010). "Management of behavioral problems in Alzheimer's disease." *International Psychogeriatrics, 22*(3), 346–372.

Gauthier, S., et al. (2022). *World Alzheimer Report: Life after diagnosis – Navigating treatment and care.* London, England: Alzheimer's Disease International.

Hölttä, E., et al. (2011). "The overlap of delirium with neuropsychiatric symptoms among patients with dementia." *American Journal of Geriatric Psychiatry, 19*(12), 1034–1041. https://doi.org/10.1097/JGP.0b013e31820dcbb6

Ismail, Z., et al. (2022). "Psychosis in Alzheimer disease — Mechanisms, genetics, and therapeutic opportunities." *Nature Reviews Neurology, 18,* 131–144. https://doi.org/10.1038/s41582-021-00597-3

Kales, H.C., et al. (2015). "Assessment and management of behavioral and psychological symptoms of dementia." *BMJ, 350,* h369.

Khachiyants, N., et al. (2011). "Sundown syndrome in persons with dementia: An update." *Psychiatry Investigation, 8*(4), 275–287. https://doi.org/10.4306/pi.2011.8.4.275

Kovach, C.R., et al. (1999). "Symptoms of discomfort in dementia and the presence of associated behaviors." *Journal of Gerontological Nursing, 25*(7), 44–53.

Kumfor, F., et al. (2022). "Examining the presence and nature of delusions in Alzheimer's disease and frontotemporal dementia syndromes." *International Journal of Geriatric Psychiatry, 37*(3), e5692. https://doi.org/10.1002/gps.5692

Livingston, G., et al. (2017). "Dementia prevention, intervention, and care: 2020 report of the Lancet Commission." *The Lancet, 390*(10113), 2673–2734.

Ma, L.Z., et al. (2022). "Time spent in outdoor light is associated with the risk of dementia: A prospective cohort study of 362,094 participants." *BMC Medicine, 20*(1), 132. https://doi.org/10.1186/s12916-022-02331-2

Morris, D.W. (2019). "Adaptive affect: The nature of anxiety and depression." *Neuropsychiatric Disease and Treatment, 15,* 3323–3326. https://doi.org/10.2147/NDT.S230491

Noetel, M., et al. (2024). "Effect of exercise for depression: Systematic review and network meta-analysis of randomised controlled trials." *BMJ, 384,* e075847. https://doi.org/10.1136/bmj-2023-075847

Orgeta, V., et al. (2022). "Psychological treatments for depression and anxiety in dementia and mild cognitive impairment." *Cochrane Database of Systematic Reviews, 4*(4), CD009125. https://doi.org/10.1002/14651858.CD009125.pub3

Patterson, C., et al. (2008). "Assessment and treatment of mental health issues in dementia: A consensus report." *American Journal of Geriatric Psychiatry, 16*(5), 421–431.

Perren, S., et al. (2006). "Caregivers' adaptation to change: The impact of increasing impairment of persons suffering from dementia on their caregivers' subjective well-being." *Aging & Mental Health, 10*(5), 539–548. https://doi.org/10.1080/13607860600637844

Steinberg, M., et al. (2006). "Risk factors for neuropsychiatric symptoms in dementia: The Cache County Study." *International Journal of Geriatric Psychiatry, 21*(9), 824–830.

Sultzer, D.L., et al. (2014). "Neurobiology of delusions, memory, and insight in Alzheimer's disease." *American Journal of Geriatric Psychiatry, 22*(11), 1346–1355. https://doi.org/10.1016/j.jagp.2013.06.005

Tetsuka, S. (2021). "Depression and dementia in older adults: A neuropsychological review." *Aging & Disease, 12*(8), 1920–1934. https://doi.org/10.14336/AD.2021.0526

Vasse, E., et al. (2010). "Factors associated with aggressive behaviour among nursing home residents with dementia: A systematic review." *International Journal of Geriatric Psychiatry, 25*(2), 143–154.

11. Maximising the good stuff

McNair, D., et al. (2011). *Light and Lighting Design for People with Dementia.* Hammond Press.

Shirsat, A., et al. (2023). "Music therapy in the treatment of dementia: A review article." *Cureus, 15*(3), e36954. https://doi.org/10.7759/cureus.36954

Acknowledgements

Nihil de nobis, sine nobis which translates to 'Nothing about us without us' has roots in Eastern European political traditions. Historically used in the 16th-century Polish-Lithuanian Commonwealth, it was a principle of governance, asserting that no decisions should be made without the consent of those affected. It is a phrase and principle that has been adopted by the disability-rights movement and embraced by other marginalised groups. Nothing about you without you is a variation often used in the context of dementia and caregiving where a more personalised, individual focus is required. I have always involved the people affected in my research and consulted with target audiences for my animations, books and even my talks to ensure that I deliver what matters most to them. This book has been enriched and improved by feedback on early drafts from people who care for or have cared for a relative with dementia. I am particularly greatful for their feedback and for sharing their personal stories and passing on wisdom from their journeys.

Jennifer Brown, I know you were concerned that your insights were too honest – you gave me exactly what I wanted - raw honest feedback. Thank you, it meant a lot to hear that what I wrote resonated with you and thank you so much for your honest insights on guilt.

Aisling Harmon – You told me that the book moved you and allowed you travel back in time to the caring moment. Thank you so much for giving me a glimpse into your life caring for your mum Carmel.

Bernadette – Thank you so much for sharing the naked truth of life as a young sole carer. I know that your words will make others feel less alone and that your wisdom will help improve the caregiving journey for readers.

Tony McIntyre – Thank you so much your words reassured me that my book was easy to understand and your comment 'I would have benefited a lot if I had read this a couple of years ago when I first started having stress caring' both moved and motivated me.

Jackie Golden – Thank you for your insightful comments. They helped to make the book more inclusive.

Diane Swann, I know you are currently a care partner so you deserve particular thanks for taking the time to read and offer your wonderful feedback on living in the moment, counting your blessings, being grateful, caring for yourself and ditching the guilt. Your advice is echoed throughout the book.

Richard Dolan – Thank you for your straight-talking. It got me thinking and editing.

Susan Crampton – What can I say? I wish I'd heard your advice before I began my own caring journey. Thank you so much for sharing your experience, I know so many readers will benefit.

Martina Nugent – Thank you for your honest feedback and for your great advice about the importance of complaining to bring about change.

Denise Monahan, thank you for giving me real life examples to elevate my text and help it resonate with readers.

Muriel Moore – I felt so happy when you told me you laughed and you cried while reading – not that I wanted to make you cry but it meant so much to know that the book resonated with you and I was honoured to learn that it brought back memories of happy, funny and tough times with your husband.

John Knox – I'd put off reading your comments because I received them as photocopied pages of handwritten script which was a little challenging to decipher but boy am I glad that I did. You moved me to tears but in a good way – your love for each other shone through. Your words and your wisdom and acceptance are inspiring. Anne was so lucky to love and be loved by you.

Máire-Anne Doyle – Thank you so much for sharing a small slice of your caring life. Thank you for sharing the wonderful advice that was shared with you about ending the day by expressing your love for your dad. Every time I read your story I get goose bumps. I too know the wise woman who gave you that advice and what a wonderful woman she is.

Joanne – You had one of the most difficult chapters of the book to read so I really appreciate your helpful feedback.

Mary Toland – Knowing you found what you read affirming gave me confidence that I was hitting the right tone – thank you.

Judy Williams, thank you so much for reading an early draft and for connecting me with all of these wonderful carers. You went above and beyond in supporting me as well as these wonderful people. The Alzheimer Society of Ireland is so lucky to have you. I can't thank you enough.

Kimberly Tully and Helen Quaid thank you both for your feedback on early drafts.

Helen-Rochford Brennan, thank you for being an inspiration and for advocating for the rights of people living with dementia. You are a warrior.

It's a given that writers thank their agents but this book genuinely would not exist without my agents Jane Graham-Maw and Amy O'Shea. I started writing this book not long after my mum passed away. I'd just finished the first draft of my first book *100 Days to a Younger Brain*. Writing about caregiving was cathartic and in some way helped me to process my grief and other complex emotions I felt not just about Mum's death but about the years that preceeded it. Margharita Solon invited me to give a talk and while there showed me around their wonderful day centre, McAuley Place. When I saw it, I cried because I felt that my mum would have loved this place and felt terrible that she didn't have somewhere as wonderful to live. Margharita said to use my experience to make sure that others that follow have a better experience. The words for the first section of this book just flowed out of me and then sat unattended while I wrote two other books. When I finished my last book Jane asked me 'what next' and I said I have a book that I am passionate about that I am not prepared to give up on despite not having a publisher for it. Over the next few months Jane, Amy and I put together a really strong proposal and they made my dream to publish this book a reality – a huge thank you to you both.

The minute I met Charlotte Croft I knew she was perfect for this book, she got it, she got me and she got my writing. It's been a dream working with you and I am so excited for *Still Me* to finally see the light of day. Thank you for not just believing in this book but for really wanting to publish it, thank you also for your incredible understanding and patience when I needed time away from writing when my son became seriously ill. I'd also like to thank Jenni Davis for copy-editing and the following people at Bloomsbury: Megan Jones, Sarah Head, Cathleen Bradford-McCormac and Ashleigh James.

Thank you Darren for surviving. Thank you Caoimhe for caring for Darren and to your parents Thomas and Winifed for supporting his recovery.

Thank you to Gavin and Jamie for just being you and for bringing fun and laughter into my life and for helping to care for Mum.

David, as always you deserve huge thanks for everything you do every single day. You were the light of my mum's life, her eyes lit up when she saw you, you did so much for her and made her so happy.

In memory of my mum Colette O'Reilly RIP 14/2/2016 and my dad who had he not died before you would have been your protector, your lover and your carer till the end. Dad was an old romantic and I've always taken solace in the fact that you were reunited with your valentine.

Index

*PLWD: People living with dementia

abusive behaviour 138–40, 144–5
   reporting 141–3
   signs of 140–1, 143–4
adaptability, care partner 203–5
adulthood, sense of 125–6
aggression and agitation 23–4, 133, 199, 212–19, 234
alarms and sensors 157–8, 256–7
alcohol consumption 222, 232
Alzheimer Society 13, 79, 94, 98, 138, 150, 154
Alzheimer's disease
   apathy 222–5
   early stage 165–7
   hallucinations and delusions 234–5, 238
   late stage 168–9
   mid stage 167–8
   physical inactivity 263
   time-shifting 243
   see also identity and independence, PLWD*
anosognosia 230
antidepressants 222–3, 229, 231
anxiety *see* depression and anxiety
apathy in PLWD* 222–8
apps, useful 105, 154, 155, 259–60
assisting *vs* doing 131–3, 148, 179, 228
assistive technology 10, 87–8, 155, 253–5
   automated prompts and reminders 256
   monitoring and tracking 157–8, 258–9
   motion-sensing devices 157, 256–7
   pill dispensers 255–6
   smart devices 257, 259–61
   'talking tiles' 258
auditory hallucinations 235, 236
avoidant coping 205–7

bathing/washing 105–6, 134
bathrooms 157, 252–3
bed-sharing 57–8
bedroom and bedtime rituals 56, 157, 180, 250
befriending services 93
behavioural and psychological symptoms of dementia (BPSD) 23–5, 78, 80, 111, 198–200, 211–12
   agitation and aggression 23–4, 133, 199, 212–19, 234
   coping strategies and practical tips 99–103, 216–19, 220–2, 227–9, 231–2, 236, 239–40, 243–4
   medication and side effects 200–1, 215, 222–3, 229, 233, 236
   recognising triggers 200, 202, 212–18, 222
   respectful responding 201–2
   sundowning 102–3, 212, 215–16, 219–22
   types of psychosis 233–44
   see also apathy in PLWD*, depression and anxiety
bereavement 202–3
boredom and dementia 133, 179
boundary setting 10, 32, 36
brain/cognitive training 184–5
brain fog 68–9
   assessment tool 70–1
   tips for clearing 84–6

breathing techniques 35, 80, 81, 102–3
bright-light therapy 58

caffeine 222, 232
care homes *see* residential care
care partner burden 25–6
   burden level questionnaire 27–9
   care activity log 26–7, 29, 32–3, 277
   challenging behaviours 24
   guilt 19–21, 33–5
   guilt-trips 21–2, 35–7
   identifying factors to address 29–30
   multitasking 85
   practical tips 30–45
   real-life stories 17–18, 23–4
   workload 22–3, 24
challenging behaviour *see* behavioural and psychological symptoms of dementia (BPSD)
childlike behaviour, understanding 125–6
Citizens Advice 98, 138
clothing issues 149, 163, 202
clutter and distractions, removing 85–6, 232
Cognitive Behavioural Therapy (CBT) 30–5
Cognitive Rehabilitation Therapy (CRT) 184, 186, 187–97
Cognitive Stimulation Therapy (CST) 12, 185–7, 227
communication, direct 149–50
   see also decision making
community activities 93
complaints, making official 141–3
control, feeling in 112, 117–18
coping, ways of
   acknowledging your feelings 104
   challenging behaviours 99–103, 105–6
   changing your perspective 101–2
   managing your stress response 102–3
   problem or solution-focused 99–101, 104–7
   real-life stories 99–103
   relaxation techniques 102–3, 207–8
   unhealthy strategies 205–7
   see also stress

decision making/opinions 135–7, 145–6, 149–50, 163, 179
Decision Support Services (Ireland) 137, 140
delegating care duties 32, 37–8, 43–4, 66, 93, 94, 104, 110
delirium 233–4, 240–2
delusions 233, 236–40
depression and anxiety
   care partner 21, 22, 46–7, 51, 52, 53–4, 74, 80, 95
   dementia, people living with 133, 171, 185, 199–200, 208–11, 215, 216, 222–3, 225, 229–32
   ways to help 231–2
diagnosis, understanding dementia (NCDs) 160, 161–2, 165
   real-life experience 159–60
   six domains of cognitive function
      complex attention 162–3

executive functions   163
  language   164
  learning and memory   163–4
  perceptual motor function   164
  social cognition   164
  see also Alzheimer's disease; early-onset/young dementia; Familial Alzheimer's; frontotemporal dementia (FTD); Lewy bodies (DLB), dementia with; mixed dementia; vascular dementia
diaries/record keeping   79–80, 99, 212, 216, 246, 248
diet and weight   60–2, 83, 84, 222, 232, 269–70
disinhibition   130, 173–4, 175–6
District/Public Health Nurses   79, 161
downplaying early stage symptoms   150–1, 178
Down's syndrome   177

early-onset/young dementia   176
education/acquiring knowledge   13, 113, 159–60, 180, 267–8
exercise/physical activity   63, 64–5, 83, 84, 104, 149, 221–2, 263–6

fall risks   156–7, 251–2
familial Alzheimer's disease   166
family and friends
  choosing the right company   96–7
  cultivating a confidant/e   98
  family conflicts   73–5
  guilt-tripping   21–2, 35–7
  importance of social connection   73, 88–9, 92–5, 96–7, 266–7
  task sharing/delegation   14, 37–8, 43–4, 66, 93, 94, 104, 110
  see also social life/leisure time
frontotemporal dementia (FTD)   160–1, 173–6, 177, 210, 238

goal setting   84, 190–2
GPs/health professionals   46, 54, 77, 138, 161, 177, 222, 229, 231, 236, 241, 254, 262
gratitude, practicing   96, 107, 271–2
group art therapy   227
guilt and guilt-tripping   19–22, 33–7

hallucinations   175, 233, 234–6
health issues, care partner   46–7, 262
  brain health   262–3, 267–8
  depression scale   53
  diet and weight   60–2, 83
  enjoying yourself   65–6
  exercise   64–5, 83
  health assessment   53–4
  health check-ups   262
  practical tips   55–60
  relationship dynamics upheaval   47–8
  sleep issues   48–53, 55–60
hearing/hearing aids/technology   87–8, 236, 270
heart health   269–70
help, asking for *see* family and friends; GPs/health professionals; support
home adaptations   248–50
  avoiding falls and trip hazards   157, 251–2
  the bathroom   157, 252–3
  the bedroom   157
  contrasting colours   250–1
  the kitchen   156, 253
  lighting   249–50, 156
  safety devices   259–60
home-care *vs* residential care   14–15, 18, 136, 138

human rights   146, 231
hydration   59–60

identification documents   153–4
identity and independence, PLWD*   11–12, 123–6, 178–80
  adult identity and infantilising   125–6, 178
  assisting *vs* doing   131–3, 148, 179, 228
  decision making and opinions   135–7, 145–6, 149–50, 179
  direct communication   149–50
  downplaying and support for early-stage symptoms   150–1, 178
  going for walks   146–8, 152–8
  risks *vs* rights   145–9, 151–8
identity, care partner loss of sense of   74
immune system   49, 84, 169
independent mental capacity advocates (IMCA)   137
irritation and anger, care partner   127–31

kitchen adaptations   253

laughter and humour   83–4
legal matters   79, 140, 150, 246, 248
Lewy bodies (DLB), dementia with   171–2, 173, 235, 238
light exposure   58–9, 221, 249–50
living well with a dementia diagnosis   183–4
  acceptance and action   245–8
  assistive technology   253–60
  enjoyment/entertainment   260–2, 264–6
  home adaptations   156–8, 248–53, 259–60
locking doors   155–6
loneliness and isolation   87, 88–91, 205
  dealing with   92–8, 266–7
  see also family and friends; social life/leisure activities; support

'me time,' protecting   32–3, 37
meal times and eating   62, 132, 148, 168–9
medication
  antidepressant   222–3, 229, 231
  managing   105, 232, 255–6
  psychotropic   200–1, 215, 229, 233
meditation and mindfulness   80, 104
memory aids   255–6
mental health, care partner   21, 22, 46–7, 51, 52, 68–71, 74, 80, 81–2, 84–6, 95
  see also depression and anxiety; stress
Mild Cognitive Impairment (MCI)   162
mixed dementia   175–6
money, access to   149
monitoring/tracking technology   154, 155, 157–8, 258–9
music therapy   227

napping   56, 221
National Health Service (NHS)   142, 185, 195–6
National Institute for Health and Care Excellence (NICE)   137, 140
negative/unhelpful thoughts, challenging   33–5, 81–2, 113–16
networks, social *see* family and friends; social life/leisure activities; support
Neurocognitive Disorders (NCDs)   162
  see also diagnosis, understanding dementia
neurologists   161
night time walking (aka wandering)   156–8, 180
non-amnestic Alzheimer's   165

INDEX | 287

occupational therapists 161, 254
online carer training 13
optimism
  cultivating 116–17
  vs pessimism 111–12
overstimulation 222

Parkinson's disease 172–3, 200–1, 223, 226
patience, importance of 127–31
Patient Advice and Liaison Service (PALS) 142
perspective, changing your 101–2, 113–16
physical health, care partner see health issues, care partner
pill organisers and dispensers 105, 255–6
positivity and reward, caring role 108–10, 247
  cultivating optimism 116–17
  enhancing capabilities by acquiring knowledge 113
  feeling in/taking control 112, 117–19
  nurturing relationships/recognising positive responses 119–20
  optimism vs pessimism 111–12
  unhelpful thoughts/shifting perspective 113–16
Power of Attorney 79, 248
preferences, documenting 246, 248
present/'in the moment,' being 81–2
private therapy 196
problem-solving 99–101, 104–7, 204
procrastination/avoidant coping 205, 206–7
professional care at home 14, 18, 32, 38, 79, 106
  choosing home care services 38–40
  helping your relative accept in-home care 40–1
psychiatrists 161
psychologists 161
psychosis 233–44

question repetition, dealing with 130

relationships, challenge of changing 47–8, 72
reminiscence therapy 227–8
residential care 15, 18, 136–7
  choosing a care home 41–2, 137
  helping your relative adjust 42–3
  recognising and reporting abusive behaviour 140–3
  restricting behaviour and sedation 146–8
restrictive measures 146–9, 155–6
risks vs rights 145–9, 151–6
routine, importance of 82–3, 157, 218–19, 222, 228, 232

safety 152–6
  agitation and aggressive behaviour 199
  assistive technology 258–60
  missing relatives 158, 180
  night time walking 156–8, 180
  see also risks vs rights
self-care 9–10, 11, 13–16, 121–2, 207, 247
  see also care partner burden; coping, ways of; family and friends; health issues, care partner; positivity and reward, caring role; stress; support
self-compassion 95
self-esteem, loss of 74
self-isolation 205
self-talk, negative see negative/unhelpful thoughts, challenging
sexual interest and behaviour 130
sleep
  bedtime rituals 56
  care partners 49–60
  choices for couples/bed-sharing 57–8

dementia patients 49, 58, 221
  and diet 50
  gender differences 51, 52
  hydration 59–60
  importance of prioritising sleep 55–6, 268
  light exposure 58–9
  napping 56, 60
SMART goals 191
smiling 270–1
social life/leisure time 73, 88–9
  asking for help 93–5, 97
  befriending services 93
  choosing the right people 96–7
  dementia, people living with 148–9, 227–8, 232, 259–61, 266–7
  hobbies 267–8
  measuring your level of perceived social support 89–91
  staying connected 92–3, 266–7
  see also friends and family; 'me' time
social media 92–3
social services/social workers 156, 161, 196
sole carers, stress and 78–80
speech and language therapists 62, 63
stress 48, 270
  affectionate physical contact 97
  assessment and log 75–8, 115
  brain fog 68–71
  care workload 22–3, 24, 67
  conflict with family 73–4
  and diet 61
  and guilt 19–22, 33–7
  juggling multiple roles 73
  loss self-esteem and sense of identity 74
  managing 79–86
  reframing stressors 115–16
  relationship with dementia patient 72
  sleep loss 52
  and sole carers 78–9
  see also coping, ways of
strokes and vascular dementia 170–1, 177
suicide risk 231
sundowning 102–3, 212, 215–16, 219–22
support
  groups/networks 45, 92, 93–4, 96, 98, 140, 153, 204, 207, 226, 229, 231
  measuring perceived social support 89–91
  organisations/services 13–14, 63, 79, 93, 94, 98, 137–8, 140–2, 150, 156, 196, 231
  professional care at home 14, 18, 32, 38–41, 79, 106, 204
  specialist roles/input 161
  supporting others - giving and receiving 96
  see also family and friends; GPs/health professionals

therapy, structured 227–8
  see also Cognitive Rehabilitation Therapy (CRT)
time-shifting 242–4
touch, affectionate human 97, 134, 178
tracking and monitoring devices 154, 155, 157–8, 258–9

urinary tract infections (UTIs) 175, 241–2

validation therapy 201–2
vascular dementia 169–71, 210–11, 238

walking (aka wandering), night time 156–8
walks, going for 146–8, 152–8, 264, 265
weight and diet see diet and weight
words and language, unfamiliar 126–7
workload, care partner see care partner burden